Follow Your Star

From Mining to Heart Transplants
– A Surgeon's Story

Terence English

authorHOUSE®

AuthorHouse™ UK Ltd.
500 Avebury Boulevard
Central Milton Keynes, MK9 2BE
www.authorhouse.co.uk
Phone: 08001974150

First published by AuthorHouse   1/25/2011.

ISBN: 978-1-4567-7131-7 (sc)
ISBN: 978-1-4567-7130-0 (dj)

Contents

FOREWORD   1

Chapter 1 Forbears and Childhood   3

Chapter 2 Rhodesia and University   24

Chapter 3 Canada and Medical School   45

Chapter 4 Surgical Training and Marriage   68

Chapter 5. Papworth Hospital and Heart Transplantation   89

Chapter 6 The General Medical Council; the Artificial Heart, and Private Practice   116

Chapter 7 Presidency of the Royal College of Surgeons (1989-1992)   144

Chapter 8 Master of St Catharine's College, (1993-2000)   174

Chapter 9 President of the BMA; the Audit Commission and Holidays (1993 – 2000)   195

Chapter 10 Remarriage and Retirement   207

APPENDIX   231

INDEX   237

About the Author   245

ACKNOWLEDGEMENTS

I am grateful to my good friend Francis Warner, Emeritus Fellow in English Literature at St. Peter's College Oxford, for having encouraged me to write this autobiography. He was then generous enough to read and comment upon each chapter as it was written. My wife, Judith, also provided helpful suggestions as the book progressed. Finally, I was especially fortunate in having the expert skills of Caroline Hill to decipher my handwriting and type the first draft, after which I was able to revise the manuscript on my computer.

FOREWORD

I have admiration for those who at an early age know what they want to do and then set about achieving this without, as they say, hesitation or deviation. However, there are others such as myself whose lives have been characterised by false starts or blind alleys, but who have generally tried to follow whatever 'star' was shining most brightly for them at any particular time, and who have not been afraid to stop and start again if a brighter one appeared on the horizon.

Looking back on my life, I can see that there have been a number of occasions when, being prepared to either change direction or take on a different challenge, has had important consequences not only for my personal circumstances but also for those around me and for determining the sort of person I have become. Once having decided on a course of action, tenacity of purpose is clearly of the utmost importance, but there is also that element of good fortune whereby one happens to be in the right place at the right time. Or to put it another way, your star beckons both at the right time and in the right direction. Whilst writing this book, I came to recognise that many such decisions resulted in a richer experience of life than might otherwise have been the case, even though they did not necessarily contribute to my eventual career. It is for this reason that "Follow your Star" seemed an appropriate title for the book.

Finally, and with some diffidence, there is an Appendix in which I include a number of aphorisms and extracts from writings that I have come across at different times of my life, and which I found sufficiently interesting to record in the journals I have kept sporadically over the years.

Chapter 1
Forbears and Childhood

A. FORBEARS

My father died when I was eighteen months old. I had a sister, Elizabeth, three years older than me but a brother, Frederick, had died in infancy a year before I was born. So my mother was left a widow at the age of 37 with two young children. My father had been a mining engineer, and at the time of his death was consulting engineer for Goldfields Development Company in Rhodesia, based in Bulawayo. My mother was from Natal but did not want to be a burden on her family and so chose to return to Johannesburg where they had started their married life. It was there that my sister and I grew up and, as we did, my mother often talked to us about our father and what a fine person he had been. She also impressed on me that I was the last male in my generation of the English family, which had been in South Africa since the early part of the 19th century. This, and wanting to know more about my father and forbears, stimulated my interest in family history on which the following account is based.

My paternal great-grandfather, Alexander English, was born in Ireland in about 1800. I was told that he initially worked in a Bank in Dublin but later moved to London where he became a glass merchant. In May 1833 he married Anne Hawthorne in Leith, Scotland, and I have the original Declaration of Marriage which reads as follows: "At Leith, in the House of John Fulton, Baltic Street, there on the Thirteenth of May, One Thousand Eight Hundred and Thirty-Three; and in the presence of John Fulton, Grain Dealer Leith; James Letham Tobacconist Leith; and Charles Hawthorn of the City of Dublin, Gentleman. I Alexander English of London, Glass Merchant, have consented and do hereby consent to acknowledge and declare myself to be the lawful Husband of Anne Hawthorne, daughter of the late Alexander Hawthorne of Dublin, Glover, after designed, and of the said Anne Hawthorne have consented and do hereby consent, acknowledge and declare myself to be the lawful wife of the said Alexander English before designed, and we do hereby declare ourselves married persons. In testimony whereof these present written upon stamped paper by John Fulton, Junior Clerk Leith – are subscribed by us – place and date foresaid – in presence of these Witnesses the said John Fulton, James Letham, and Charles Hawthorne."

The Declaration, which has a Five Shilling stamp on it is in a fine state of preservation and is signed by the married couple and the three witnesses.

After their marriage they lived in Maida Vale in London where their first child, Jane Elizabeth, was born. Anne's youngest sister, Jane Hawthorne, had come to London with them and later that year, and for no clear reason that I can determine, they all set sail for South Africa, landing in Cape Town in early 1835. It must have been a difficult voyage, lasting several months and with Anne pregnant with her second child, Anna Maria, who was born in Cape Town in May of that year.

Initially they lived in Bouquet Street where my grandfather, William Henry English, was born on 26th May 1837, the year that Queen Victoria came to the throne. There followed two children who died in infancy, and then Arthur Wellesley (29th January 1842); Emily Catherine (13th November 1843) and Frederick Alexander (20th August 1845). Later they moved to an old Dutch house on the side of Signal Hill at Green Point which they called "Sweet Home" and which became the centre of their large and expanding family. My great-grandfather obtained employment with the Cape of Good Hope Bank, where he subsequently rose to Chief Accountant. My great-grandmother was well educated and the children received all their primary education at home.

I have in my possession "Recollections of the Dear House at Green Point" given to me by my father's cousin, Jean Gordon, which she wrote shortly before her death in 1952. She was the last member of the family to live there and the first two paragraphs read as follows:

"The household consisted at that time (late-1870s) of Grandpappa and Grandmamma, Uncle Arthur the second son a bachelor; Marie and Louis Paré, children of Anna and Victor Paré; Ellen and Charlotte Little, daughters of Jane, the eldest daughter who had married Michael Little in India and then died during the Mutiny in 1857; my mother Emily Gordon, my sister Isoline and myself, and Ernest, the son of Anna and Michael Little whom my mother adopted when his mother died of dysentery in India when he was three months old. Five different families all at home under the roof of the dear old grandparents who had large hearts. The eldest son William was a magistrate in Humansdorp and Fred, the youngest, was farming in Victoria West.

Grandmama was a tall, graceful woman with a sweet face. She was a good classical scholar and knew Italian and French well. None of the children or grandchildren went to school; she educated them all as she had a first-class girls' finishing school with visiting masters. When William and Arthur went to the South African College, the head (I think it was Sir Langham Dale, but I'm not sure) wrote to her and said he wished all his pupils were as well grounded in the classics as her sons".

I also have in my possession a diary kept by my grandfather from 1860 to 1865 whilst he was still living at home. This recounts his activities and lists his daily expenditure including how much he spent on "baccy", his reading habits, and how often he played chess with his father. He belonged to the Cape Town Mutual Improvement Society and I have a copy of his contribution to a debate on "Are the English or Scotch the more patriotic people?" This took place on 18th December 1857 when he was twenty years old and it seems the decision came down in favour of the English. The following year he joined the Colonial Secretary's Department as a clerk and then progressed to

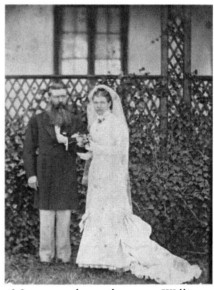

My paternal grandparents, William English and Katherine Human on their wedding day (29 September 1880)

1st Clerk to the Secretary of Native Affairs before being appointed Clerk to the Civil Commissioner in East London in 1873. Four years later he became Civil Commissioner and Resident Magistrate in Humansdorp and it was there that he met and married my grandmother, Katherine Elizabeth Human in 1880. He was then 43 and she twenty years his junior and I have a fascinating collection of letters he wrote during his courtship. To start with these are very formal, an example of which follows:

"My dear Miss Human, I had an interview with your father this morning and it is my great happiness to be able to say that I have his sanction to ask you to be my dear wife.

I should have come out today but am prevented by office work of the most urgent nature. I hope and expect to see you tomorrow either here or at Sandrift as I shall call on my way home.

I wish I had a "forget me not" to enclose – in its absence I send you a sprig of myrtle. Did you notice that there was a bit of that shrub in a small bouquet I gave you many Sundays ago?

Yours very sincerely,

W.H. English"

Later the correspondence becomes more tender, romantic and even playful as evidenced

by this note:

"To Her Majesty, Queen Katherine,

The Petition of William Henry Dutton English of Humansdorp:

That your Petitioner is very desirous of approaching Your Majesty, and therefore prays that Your

Majesty will deign to inform Petitioner at what hour today Your Majesty will hold Court under the Fig Tree.

And your Petitioner as in duty bound will ever pray (and fight),

      W.H. English"

And then also:

"My darling Katie,

I am "wasting paper" and Government time to tell you what I have thought fifty times during the last half hour, namely that you are a dear sweet pet, dearer to me every time I see you, that is if the utmost limit of love has not already been reached by now.

You ought to be glad that I was smoking when we were in the garden just now or I should have hugged and kissed you without mercy before any and everyone.

In great haste,

Your most devoted, William.

The year after their marriage he was transferred to Robertson as Civil Commissioner and Resident Magistrate and it was there that they acquired "Druid's Lodge", a large old farmhouse with extensive grounds in the centre of the town. During the next seven years their first five children were born: Maud, Elzabe, Arthur (my father, born 22nd November 1884), Jessie and Violet. In 1890 he was again transferred, this time to Victoria West, at which time he was earning £600 a year. Their two youngest sons Fred and Henry were born there. In 1895 he asked to be released from duty on health grounds and they returned to Robertson where he spent just

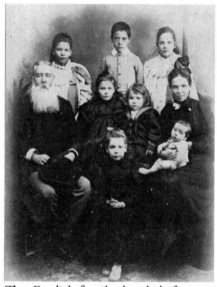

The English family shortly before my grandfather's death – my father is top centre

over a year in retirement before his death at the age of 59 in 1896. This left Katherine a widow at the early age of 39 with seven young children to bring up.

My maternal grandmother was of the sixth generation of Humans to have lived in the Cape. The first, Johann Human of Solingen, had arrived in 1703 as a soldier of the Dutch East India Company and later became Servant of the Governor, William Adriaan van der Stel who had succeeded his father Simon van der Stel as Governor in 1699. Johann became a "Free Burgher" in 1710 and two years later married Lysbeth Vion ("of the Cape"). The next two generations remained in Stellenbosch but in

1836 the family moved further inland, as part of the Great Trek by the Dutch community to get away from British colonial rule, the Cape having been ceded to Britain in 1806 after the Napoleonic wars. They farmed in an area not far from what is now Port Elizabeth which became known as Humansdorp after Matthys Gerhardus Human (1798-1875) who had given land on which to build a church for the expanding community in 1849. A photograph of this stern-looking gentleman – my maternal great-great-grandfather - resides in the vestry of the Dutch Reformed Church in Humansdorp.

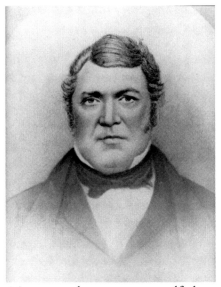

My maternal great-great grandfather, Matthys Gerhardus Human

This is where, on the farm Sandrift, my grandmother grew up, being one of four children of Jurie Johannes Human. She must have been an adventurous young woman because in her early " twenties" she did two long journeys by ox wagon, one with her uncle and the other with her father. She kept a brief daily record during the first of these, which lasted from 15ᵗʰ March to 28ᵗʰ August, and in it she records the numerous farms they visited and the friends and relations they met on their long journey up to the Transvaal and back.

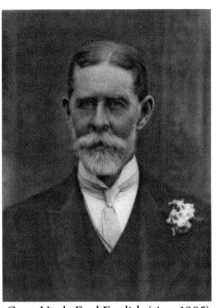

Great Uncle Fred English (circa 1905)

After my grandfather's death she remained in Robertson where she brought up her seven children. I only learned late in life how generous my grandfather's younger brother, Great Uncle Fred, was during this time. Fred English had made his fortune in the diamond and gold fields of Kimberley and Johannesburg and was then living in Addington Palace near Croydon. He and his wife Kitty (nee Devenish) had no children and perhaps this contributed to the great generosity towards his brother's family, for not only did he arrange for my grandmother to receive a grant of £300 p.a. but he also paid for the three eldest children to have their education in England. Maud and Elzabe went to Cheltenham Ladies' College and my father first to Tonbridge and then to the Royal School of Mines. They spent their holidays at Addington and I believe the younger children would have been similarly treated, had not Uncle Fred died in 1909. Kitty remained in England, first at Addington and later at Pickhurst Manor in Hayes, Kent. She then returned to South Africa in 1924 when she bought and restored the beautiful wine estate of "Lanzerac" near Stellenbosch.

My grandmother became a well-known figure in Robertson spending the remaining 28 years of her life there after my grandfather's death. She was always proud of the fact that her three sons had fought throughout the Great War, and remarkably that all had survived, and that two of them, my father and Fred, had received the Military Cross. Three of the four daughters remained spinsters, two of them becoming teachers. The youngest, Violet, was my godmother and as a boy I loved listening to accounts of her adventures in India and Rhodesia. When she retired she returned to "Druid's Lodge" and lived there until her death in 1976.

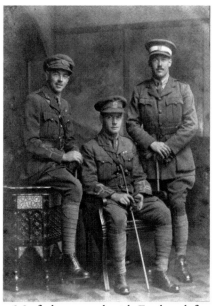

My father seated with Fred on left and Henry standing, in 1916

I had bought the property some years earlier in order that the remaining siblings could benefit from their inheritance, as although all of them were equal beneficiaries, my grandmother's Will decreed that any unmarried members of the family should be allowed to live there free of charge until their death. However, soon after Violet died the Municipality expropriated the property for a paltry sum and then built eleven houses on the greater part of the land. The house itself was saved from demolition and now houses the Robertson Museum, in which there is a lot of material from the long residence of my father's family, including some beautiful lace work by my aunts.

My mother's family also had a long history in South Africa. Her paternal grandfather was part of a group of immigrants from the East Riding of Yorkshire who set sail for Natal on the good ship "Haidee" in 1850. This was just five years after the Boer republic of "Natalia" had been annexed by Britain and was part of a Colonial Office scheme of making land bounties to the promoters of emigration, applicable to co-operative parties as well as companies. The Natal party had been recruited through the energy and optimism of a handful of substantial tenant farmers. Two men were prominent in this. Henry Boast was from North Dalton and my great-grandfather Benjamin Lund (b. 15th April 1821) from Sheriff Hutton. A small committee was formed that toured the East and North Ridings enlisting the interest of small farmers in the new colony of Natal and collecting passage money from those who had made up their minds. Boast and Lund were eventually able to deposit £2,000 with the Colonial and Land Emigration Commissioners, thereby entitling them to make their own arrangements for the passage. They proposed to bear all expenses on a joint basis, distributing any profits that might emerge later.

Unfortunately the first ship they contracted to transport the party to Port Natal was pronounced unseaworthy. By this time the prospective emigrants were flocking into Hull in readiness for their departure and although a substitute ship was provided, namely the three-master "Haidee", the delay meant that it became necessary to distribute

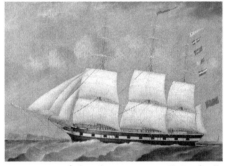

Painting of the three-master "Haidee"

rations and allowances to those emigrants who were without means. An action in the magistrates' court established that Boast was liable at law to furnish these allowances caused by the delay in sailing. He accomplished this but then died at the early age of 34 before the "Haidee" was ready to sail. However, the Hull folk, suffering as they were from the depression of the time, rallied round the future Natal colonists and the Mayor opened a relief fund for their assistance.

The ship left Hull on 10th July 1850 and arrived off Port Natal on 7th October with 246 emigrants on board. The land purchased for their settlement was some 30 miles from Pietermaritzburg and here the small village of York was quickly established. Most of the settlers were farmers and despite difficult conditions they soon began to make a success in their new environment. York was not a particularly suitable area for growing crops and with time many spread out into the more fertile districts of the midlands of Natal.

A year after their arrival, Benjamin Lund married Jane Plummer at York on 6th August 1851. Jane and her brother and sister had also been passengers on the ship, during which time she kept an interesting diary, excepts of which were published in a document celebrating the 150th Anniversary of the arrival of the Haidee Settlers held in Natal on 7th October 2000. During the next sixteen years Benjamin and Jane had two daughters and five sons of whom my grandfather, Charles Luke Lund (b. 21st March 1863), was the second youngest. Benjamin died by drowning in 1886 and Jane died later the same year. My grandfather apparently had little formal education but with ability

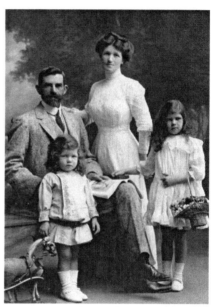

My maternal grandparents Charles Lund and Evelyn Stewart with my mother and Doreen (circa 1900).

and determination he became a successful farmer. With the coming of the Union of South Africa in 1910 he was elected to the Provincial Council, serving on the Executive Committee for many years. He was interested in education and became a member of the Governing Bodies of St Anne's and Hilton College where his three sons and three daughters went to school.

On 1st June 1894 he married Evelyn Stewart and their first home was the farm "Malden", situated below Hilton where my mother and Doreen were born. Later they acquired "Clifton" which subsequently became part of Hilton College Estate and which I remember passing on cross-country runs when I was a schoolboy. Then in 1922 he bought the lovely farm "Montrose" near Merrivale, which the eldest son, Guy, inherited after my grandfather's sudden death from a stroke on 17th October 1923 and where, later, all our family would gather for Christmas.

My mother, Mavis Eleanor Lund, was the eldest of the six children, having been born on 1st April 1896, and after leaving St Anne's, where she was Head Girl in her last year, she trained as a nurse in Johannesburg and it was there that she met and married my father in 1923. Her five siblings, Doreen, Guy, Alfred, Ruth and Max mostly had large families, providing me with seventeen first cousins of whom I became very fond and, as will be seen later, my Uncle Max who was a surgeon became a great influence in my life. In summary, I believe my grandfather Lund was a remarkable man and for both its general and historical interest I include "An Appreciation" written by William Falcon, Headmaster of Hilton College at the time of his death.

THE LATE MR. C.L. LUND, M.P.C., J.P. died 17.10.23

To every man at times, as he gazes back over the years, comes the vision of Travellers crossing the Great Divide. One by one in an endless stream he sees them pass – the aged man, who has fulfilled his alloted span, the child in the first flush of early youth, young men and maidens, men in the full vigour of manhood, and tender babes – till the mind is numbed in wonder at the inscrutable ways of God.

With such wonder most of us must have met the first shock of the passing of Charles L. Lund. He had been so recently among us, the picture of health and vigour, so full of life and energy. Throughout the Midlands, and the Northlands of Natal, who did not know the tall, well-knit figure, the bronzed alert face, the cheery word, the kindly smile. At agricultural meetings, at church bazaars, at political and social gatherings, wherever in short men do congregate, no figure more familiar, no face more welcome!

His life was one that well may be a beacon of hope, and an inspiration to many a Natal boy. Born in this country of sturdy Yorkshire stock, he had few of the advantages of early education 60 years ago which are now within the reach of every boy, but he had what is better still, grit and determination and boundless energy. With these he carved a road to success for himself, and after 20 years of strenuous work he was known as one of the most successful and progressive farmers in the Midlands of Natal.

With the coming of Union he was invited to stand for the Umgeni Division of the Provincial Council. Though naturally of a somewhat shy and retiring disposition, his high sense of duty and his great public spirit overrode all personal inclinations. The election was won with ease, and he continued to represent the division until his death. For four years he was a member of the Executive Council, and during that period he spent much of his time travelling about the Province to gain a closer knowledge of the outlying districts. It was characteristic of the man that he accepted no office or trust without giving to it of the best that was in him, at whatever sacrifice of time and money. A good politician he never was, and never could have been. His whole nature would have revolted against the thraldom of the party system; he could no more have voted against his convictions than he would have done evil that good might come of it. For him there was but one course open at all times, and that was loyalty to his own conscience.

He never adopted a policy because it was the popular one. On every question he brought to bear a mind that was singularly clear and logical, tempered by a heart that was full of sympathy with his fellow-men; and while we often find him on the losing side, we also find that time has generally vindicated his views.

He had no faith in the maxim that speech is given to man to hide his thoughts, and so in business and in politics, as in all the affairs of life, his transparent honesty and sincerity won for him the respect of all with whom he came in touch.

His interest in education was great. He read much and pondered deeply on the problems of this much debated matter, and his views were fundamentally very sound. For many years he was a member of the Governing Bodies of St. Anne's College and of Hilton College, and did valuable service to both these institutions, sparing neither time nor trouble in furthering their interests. Few men have given so freely of valuable time or supported so generously the cause of education. His wise counsel and kindly encouragement will be sadly missed.

In private life his kindness and generosity were unbounded. Many a young man owes to Mr. Lund his chance of making good; no genuine supplicant appealed to him in vain for a helping hand.

"Call no man happy until a happy death has closed a happy life" was the reply of the Ancient Sage to the millionaire king of old, who wondered why he, with all his power and wealth, had not received the verdict as the happiest of all men.

Well may we call you happy, Charles Lund! It is not for you that we must grieve, but for the loving sharer in all your toil and all your joys, for the stalwart sons and splendid daughters who without you feel the whole world a void till Time, the Healer, shall soften the poignancy of their grief, and fill the aching void with the noble memory. What more could your dearest friend wish you than you have attained! A life full of strenuous work and great accomplishment; the love and gratitude of your own dear ones; the affection of your friends; the respect and esteem of all your fellow-men; and at the last – no dimming of the eye, no enfeebling of the frame, in the full power of your manhood, and in the pride of an upright and stainless life you have ridden out into the Unknown to face your Maker, dauntless and unafraid.

W. FALCON,
Headmaster, Hilton College

October 1923

I know less about my maternal grandmother than my other grandparents. She was born Evelyn Lizzie Stewart in Scotland on 28th November 1872 and was one of nine children. Soon afterwards the family emigrated to South Africa and settled in Swaziland. The parents died when the children were still quite young. However, the brothers supported their four sisters through St Anne's boarding school near Hilton. My grandmother died in 1935 so I have no recollection of her but I did get to know and have clear memories of two of her sisters, Aunt Bea and Aunt Mabs. They were both very short, as was my grandmother, and very 'proper'. Bea married Harold Nicholson, who had been helped personally along the way by my grandfather Lund. They lost two sons in the First World War and the surviving son was said to be married and living in a mud hut somewhere in Swaziland. Their daughter Eileen married a farmer in Natal and their son, Owen, became a good friend of mine. Mabs married "Wattie" Boast and they lived in Pigs Peak, a delightful village situated in the mountainous area of Swaziland near the Transvaal border. They had three daughters, Betty, Pam and Eve all of whom were educated at St Anne's with Mabs's brother, Bert, paying the bills.

Bert and his four brothers, Jamie, Val, Malcolm and Jack seemed to have lived an adventurous and sometimes irresponsible life in Swaziland. They were very musical and drank heavily and there were stories of a number of illegitimate black children who called themselves 'Stewarts'. Their sons were also a wild lot and as a boy I used to look forward to their occasional visits to Johannesburg for family events, when there would be much music, drinking and misbehaviour before they returned to Swaziland. So, like many South Africans, I am the product of a mixture of nationalities that in my case include Irish, Afrikaans, Yorkshire and Scottish elements, all of which must have had some influence in contributing to make me what I am.

My Father. Arthur Alexander English.

After completing his training at the Royal School of Mines in London my father, Arthur English, returned to South Africa in 1907 and began his mining career in Johannesburg. He was employed by Consolidated Gold Fields of South Africa Limited, which Cecil Rhodes had founded when gold had been discovered on the Witwatersrand in 1886. He gained his early experience on the Robinson Deep Mine and had progressed to Mine Captain by the time the First World War broke out. He immediately enlisted in the Imperial Light Horse and fought in German South West Africa where he served until September 1915, by which time the Germans had been defeated.

He then travelled to England and with his mining experience joined a Tunnelling Company of the Royal Engineers. After two years of what must have been dangerous and difficult work he put in for a transfer to the Royal Flying Corps and after the necessary training returned to France in September 1917. A month later he was lucky to survive after being shot down in an air battle over the trenches, during which he sustained a severe abdominal bullet wound. However, he was able to return to France in early 1918 and ended the war as senior pilot in his flight of six machines belonging to 101st Squadron. He had won the Military Cross during his service as a tunneller and for his role in the Air Force he was mentioned in a Despatch from Field Marshall Sir Douglas Haig dated 16th March 1919 and signed by Winston Churchill, Secretary of State for War. This and his war medals are amongst my treasured possessions.

After the War he returned to Johannesburg where he resumed his mining career. He became first Underground Manager and then Manager of Sub-Nigel Mine by the time of his marriage to my mother in 1923. However, not long after this he was diagnosed as having silicosis, or Miner's phthisis as it was known on the Rand. I learned subsequently that at that time, because of bad ventilation and poor dust control in the deep gold mines, the average duration between exposure to working underground and contracting the disease was about 10 years. This was true for my father, and to exacerbate matters his lungs had already suffered as a result of being gassed during the War.

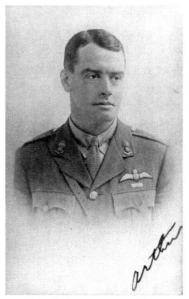

My father in 1917, after transferring to the RFC.

This meant that he could no longer continue working underground so he was sent first to Lydenburg in the Eastern Transvaal where Gold Fields were developing a platinum mine and then in 1928 became Manager of Waterval Platinum mines at Rustenburg. From there he had a short spell as consulting engineer for Gold Fields in Rhodesia before his untimely death in February 1934 at the age of 49 from respiratory failure.

B. CHILDHOOD

As mentioned, after my father's death my mother decided to settle in Johannesburg. Earliest memories are of us living in a boarding house with my mother not

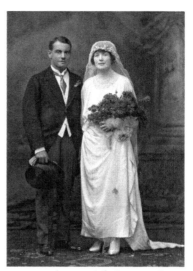

My mother and father on their wedding day (1 February 1923)

being well. However, within eighteen months she was able to buy a pleasant house with a run-down garden in Loch Avenue in Parktown, about four miles from the centre of the city. This provided us with a very happy home for the next eighteen years. My mother was a keen gardener and during the ensuing years derived much pleasure from terracing and transforming the garden into one of beauty, though inevitably never entirely to her satisfaction.

Although we were not well off we had two servants who both lived on site. Jim, who came from Malawi with a permit to work in South Africa, helped in the garden and in numerous other ways. Angelina cooked and did some of the housework. While with us she had a son and baby Ephraim soon became part of the family. Her husband, Enoch, who by law was not allowed to live on the property because he was not employed by us, was the lead pianist in a Black band called "The Golden City Swingsters". On one occasion Elizabeth and I managed to persuade him to give us a performance while our mother was out. This was enjoyed hugely until my mother's unexpected return brought proceedings to an abrupt and embarrassing halt.

With my mother's capacity for friendship and sympathy for all and sundry, we seemed to have numerous visitors and friends or family to stay. Her sister, my Aunt Doreen, was widowed in 1940 when her husband Desmond, who was a pilot, died in an air crash in East Africa. She and my mother had always been close and so Doreen came to live not far from us and her two daughters, Fay and Corinne, became more like sisters to me than cousins. Of all the visitors, one whom my sister and I came to view with suspicion was the vicar of our local church, Mr Cardrass-Grant. We felt he was paying too much attention to our mother and might wish to marry her whereas we wanted to keep her to ourselves. I doubt that there was ever any romantic inclination on either side, certainly not on our mother's, and happily our fears proved to be groundless.

After a year at Miss Cherry's kindergarten at the bottom of Loch Avenue I was sent to Parktown Preparatory School for boys. We had a smart uniform but the teaching was poor and it remains memorable only for one event. This was when I discovered a box of what I thought were chocolates in my mother's bathroom cabinet. In fact they were Brooklax, a powerful laxative. Anyway I took them to school and on arrival generously distributed them to a large number of my friends. The result by mid-morning was dramatic with small boys running repeatedly to the lavatories. The Headmaster, Mr Hadland, was furious and when he found out that I was the culprit I had a terrible dressing-down in front of the whole school.

At the age of ten my mother decided to send me as a boarder to Cordwallis School. This was in Pietermaritzburg, 300 miles and an overnight train journey away. I am not sure of her reason for this but suspect that because of her great love for me she was worried that she might become over-protective. Also perhaps because of the very feminine environment in which I was living, she may have thought that it would be to my advantage to be on my own for more of the year. Furthermore, as my cousin Michael Shaw, with whom I had become good friends was already there, I would be able to spend some of the exeats on his farm in the Karkloof with my Aunt Ruthie and Uncle Gower.

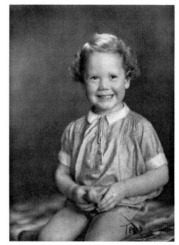

Aged 4, ready for kindergarten.

Early memories are somewhat scant but I do remember the excitement of the long overnight train journey from Johannesburg followed by a long hot walk from Pietermaritzburg station up Town Hill to the school. As new boys we slept on the covered verandah outside the dormitories for most of the year and on Sundays we had to wear Eton collars for Chapel which were wholly unsuitable at any time and particularly during the hot summer months. The teaching was for the most part excellent and the two Penningtons, Maurice and Gerald, stood out as everything good prep-school masters should be. The Headmaster, Mr Besant, was a dignified grey eminence in the background and his daughter, Diana, taught us mathematics. I don't think I can blame her for my first maths report when I went to Hilton which read simply: "His maths are but weak", but I can thank her for an entirely unexpected letter 50 years later when she wrote from Devon congratulating me on the award of my knighthood! Miss Lahee was a young attractive Afrikaans teacher and I can recall her weeping once when she bumped into me after I had been beaten up in a fight. These fights used to take place behind a shed somewhere in the grounds late on a Saturday afternoon. This meant that if you were challenged to a fight say on a Monday, you had to keep your grudge going for five days before combat commenced. Such contests usually drew an interested and vociferous crowd of onlookers, backing one or other of the combatants. However, I remember very little bullying by older boys.

Sport was important and I remember being envious of what a gifted all-round sportsman my cousin Michael Shaw was, who in our last year captained both the 1st XV and the 1st XI. I enjoyed the rugby and in the Summary of the 1st XV players Maurice Pennington wrote: "TAH English (Colours). Wing. Excellent in defence. A determined runner with a good swerve. Pity he is not faster."

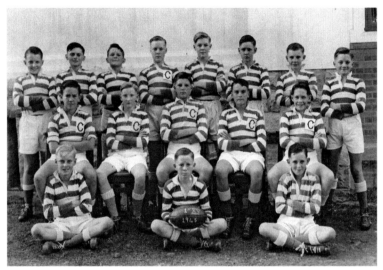

Cordwallis 1st XV 1945 – seated far right.

This proved to be somewhat prophetic because later at Hilton, when my lack of speed became more apparent, I changed position to wing-forward. The War came to an end in 1945 during my last year and VE Day was celebrated by a school holiday when we all went up to the top of Town Hill for a splendid picnic. By the end of the year it was time to leave Cordwallis and continue my education at Hilton College, with most of my friends including Michael Shaw going on to Michaelhouse.

Hilton had been established in 1872 as a boarding school for farmers' sons but is now one of the top academic schools in South Africa. It is situated on an estate of 2,000 acres in the Midlands of Natal with the school occupying a beautiful position overlooking the Umgeni river valley with the mountains of Karkloof in the distance. The main building and individual boarding houses are painted white in traditional Cape Dutch style and there is a fine stone chapel. When I last visited it two years ago I could not imagine many schools in the world with finer buildings and playing fields and a more perfect setting.

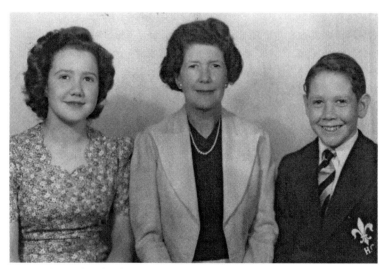

My mother, Elizabeth and me during my first year at Hilton. (1946)

The Lunds had a long association with the school, my grandfather having been a governor and my three uncles and their sons all having attended it. It is unusual in its governance in that the school is owned and governed by its Old Boys. This, as might be expected, led to very traditional attitudes and practices which were resistant to change and which remained prevalent when I was there. For example, the day would start at 6.30am in summer and 7am in winter with the ringing of the huge slave bell. This would result in 300 sleepy boys forming up on the front lawn for ten minutes of gymnastics. Then back to our respective houses for a cold plunge after which we went to first lesson. Only then did we get breakfast, which was followed by Chapel and then lessons all morning with a short break for tea. Afternoons were given to sport; rugby during winter and cricket and hockey in summer. If it was raining there would be a cross-country run and there were also regular sessions in the gym. These were conducted by an extremely fit seventy-plus year old gym-master called "Pabby" Bould (after his initials P.A.B.). He had served in the Merchant Navy and had a rich turn of phrase, one of his favourites being, if you were performing poorly, to clasp your biceps and shout: "Soft as Minnie's tits, Man. Soft as Minnie's tits!" Minnie being his diminutive wife.

The standard of sport at Hilton has always been very high and something the school is proud of. Indeed in my time there were no fewer than four future international rugby players (Paul Johnston, Brian Pfaff, Nick Labuschagne and Clive Ulyatt) and three future Springbok cricketers

(John Waite, Roy McLean and Michael Melle) in the school. I was keen on rugby but with competition as it was I never progressed beyond the 3rd XV. I suspect one reason for this was that I was rather late maturing physically compared with many of the senior boys. However, the teaching was for the most part excellent and I was pleased to get a 1st Class Matric, although disappointed that there were no distinctions amongst the seven subjects that I sat.

Discipline was rigorous and there was lots of corporal punishment, both by prefects who carried great power, and by masters. I remember returning home during my first year and my mother bursting into tears when she happened to see the black and blue bruises across my behind. The last caning I had was when I had the dubious distinction of being caned as a prefect by the Headmaster, which was a result of the following. I was never very good at cricket and the 3rd XI, of which I was a member, was coached by a very short rather disagreeable master named Mr Corbett. During practice one afternoon I had been bowling at him and to my chagrin he was treating this with disdain and hitting my balls all over the ground. I finally sent down what I thought was a particularly good one only for this to be dispatched in similar fashion. As I walked away I muttered: "That was a very big hit for a very little man", which unfortunately Mr Corbett heard and took great exception to. He duly reported me to the Headmaster who declared that he had no option but to punish my insolence by giving me six-of-the-best. This had awkward consequences as for some weeks I had to take my showers surreptitiously and at a different time from the younger boys in our House, as I did not want them to see the state of my behind.

It was this archaic prefectorial system that led indirectly to the Headmaster's resignation three years after I left the school. Terence Mansergh had been Headmaster during my first two years and was recognised as one of Hilton's great headmasters. In his youth he had captained Cambridge and England at hockey and was a master at Wellington before coming to Hilton in 1934. He had managed throughout the War with a diminished staff under difficult circumstances and after his long and selfless service was ready for retirement. Being junior I saw little of him but remember him as a man of natural dignity and authority. On his retirement the Governors appointed John Pateman as his successor. He was then thirty-four and had been housemaster at Loretto School in Scotland for short periods before and after his war service. Inevitably with his youth and lack of experience of South Africa the challenge must have been formidable. All seemed to go well during the first few years, apart from many of the senior boys falling in love with his beautiful wife Jean! I liked and admired him and despite the earlier punishment referred to he gave me a generous final year report. However, the year after I left, the school became involved in a long and highly publicised legal battle brought by a parent whose son had been "brushed" by a prefect. It was eventually settled in favour of the school in the Appellate Division of the Supreme Court but Pateman's authority had clearly been damaged. Two years later the end came when 200 boys in the Upper School walked out and spent the night in the nearby plantations. The next morning they were induced to return by the Second Master, after which they presented a list of grievances to the Vice-Chairman of Governors who had arrived the same day to investigate the incident in the absence of the Chairman overseas. Many of their complaints centred on the style of the Headmaster's leadership and his relationship with senior boys including the prefects. Pateman made concessions but the final blow occurred ten days later when a letter was sent to the Chairman of Governors, signed by every member of staff except one, which concluded: "We feel that we can confidently state that we have stood by the Headmaster very firmly indeed, but we cannot contemplate the future of Hilton College under him with anything but the gravest misgivings". Pateman had no option but to resign and left after a dignified report on his last Speech Day. Sadly he never taught again. He returned to England and joined the London Office of Anglo American where I went to see him soon after I arrived in England. Thereafter we would meet occasionally and after a while and until his death he occasionally came to the annual dinners put on by the London Hiltonian Old Boys' Society. What a sad professional failure to have had to live with.

The fortunes of the school were quickly restored by the appointment for four years of the retiring Headmaster of Maritzburg College, John William Hudson. He was sixty at the time and provided the firm hand and, most of all, the experience that was needed to regain the confidence of staff and boys and set a clear course for his successor to embark on. And now, fifty years later, as already mentioned, Hilton has for some time been one of the pre-eminent schools in South Africa. Looking back on my time there I have mixed feelings. I loved the Sundays when, after Chapel, we would be issued with sandwiches and told not to return to the school grounds until 6 pm. During this time one was free to roam the estate, go bird-watching, swim in the Umgeni river, or pursue any other outdoor activity that took your fancy as long as you remained within the 2000 acres of land owned by the school. And I believe part of my love of the outdoors stems from this experience. I received a good broad education for which I was grateful but I made few good friends and never felt entirely at ease with my surroundings. Superficially this may not have been apparent and I can remember how pleased my mother was when she made one of her rare visits to the school and was told by my housemaster, John Harker, that he could usually tell when a boy did not have a father but that this had not been the case with me. Overall, I have to conclude that, however difficult it was at times, the lessons I learned there stood me in good stead in later life.

Chapter 2
Rhodesia and University

Towards the end of my last term at Hilton I received a letter from my sister Elizabeth, wishing me well for the matriculation examination I was about to sit and finishing with the following: "How would you like to have a job in an engineering firm for a year before you start at University? It's the next best to being a sailor, and I know I would have preferred to work for a year before my degree, and gone there as an adult instead of a school kid. It's just a suggestion to think over when you've got a minute to spare, which I expect you haven't."

So when my school days ended and I had returned home, I began to follow up her suggestion. I had been due to start a four- year BSc course in civil engineering at Witwatersrand University in Johannesburg at the beginning of the academic year in February. I would have chosen mining engineering in order to follow in my father's footsteps but understandably my mother was very much against this having seen my father die at an early age from silicosis. In any event, the university was prepared to allow me to defer entry for a year, and after various investigations I managed to secure a job for the year with Cementation Company (Africa) Ltd. Cementation had made their reputation by constructing the tunnel under the Mersey between Liverpool and Birkenhead. Their main expertise lay in the process of sealing porous rock formations by first drilling holes into the rock and then pumping in liquid cement under pressure to infiltrate the cracks and crevices in the rock rendering it impermeable to water. There was a considerable demand for this in the deep gold mines of the Witwatersrand, or the Rand, as it was frequently known by those living in Johannesburg.

However, I was to be sent on a contract they had won in Rhodesia as part of a large dam that was to be built some 20 miles south of what was then

Salisbury, now Harare. The dam in the Hunyani River was planned to supply the water needs of Greater Salisbury for 50 years and would result in a lake nine miles long and 5000 acres in extent, which would also provide a pleasure resort for the public. It was to be the first major composite earth-rockfill dam to be built in Southern Africa. The main contractor for the project was a firm called Clifford Harris (Rhodesia) Ltd and Cementation's contract related to sealing the banded ironstone formation bordering the concrete spillway of the dam.

The managing director of Cementation in the head office in Johannesburg was a man called Crawhall and he agreed to take me on for a year as work experience towards my engineering degree. I was duly signed on in mid-January to start on the munificent salary of £2 per month, with an additional cost of living allowance of £8 per month. So it was that, having recently turned 17, I was about to embark on a very different way of life from what I had experienced until then. However, I looked forward to this with enthusiasm and relished the thought of working with men from different backgrounds to my own and with a lot to learn about manhood.

I initially spent a few days at the Company's workshop in Johannesburg, getting to know the foreman in charge of our contract, Johnny Geldenhuys, and the two men who were to drive the rather old 5 ton Bedford truck to Rhodesia. This was heavily loaded with machinery and camping equipment and I received permission to load my shotgun and my ancient 1936 BSA motorcycle onto the back. Johnny Geldenhuys was to drive ahead of us with his wife and we were to follow. My two companions were Piet van Rensburg, an immensely strong Afrikaner and Jim Pearson, a rather weedy-looking recent immigrant from England. They took an instant dislike to each other. The cab of the truck was designed with only two seats, so I opted to ride on the back with the equipment and did so through most of the eventful 800 mile journey which followed.

We were two days late in starting and then having finally got away at noon instead of 8am as planned, the truck broke down on the outskirts of Johannesburg and we had to be towed ignominiously back to the works. Two days later we made another late start, reaching Warmbaths, about 100 miles north of Johannesburg where we spent the night. The next morning we were up at 4am and away before sunrise. Later in the morning I was joined in the back of the truck by two tramps who Piet had decided to give a lift to. That night we had a comfortable evening at the Punch Bowl Inn not far from the Rhodesian border at Beit Bridge, which we passed through the next day without event. Once inside Rhodesia the weather changed and we encountered intermittent rain that meant I spent time in the cab lodged between Piet and Jim who spent much of the time arguing. The roads also deteriorated so we made slow progress with two further overnight stops before the truck finally broke down 20 miles short of our destination. However, we had the luxury of being provided with hotel accommodation in Salisbury that night before finally arriving at our temporary campsite at Hunyani Poort six days after leaving Johannesburg.

I had no specific duties to start with, being very much an odd job man looking after the pumps and machinery and helping to prepare the permanent tented campsite, closer to where our work would be. Early in February two more Afrikaners joined us. Hennie Jansen was to be in charge of the wagon-drilling and Sarel De Beer responsible for the pumps that drove cement into the ground via the holes once these had been drilled. Sarel was a colourful character with a past history of illicit diamond buying. We all got on reasonably well and I was surprised and pleased when Piet asked me to be his Best Man at his wedding in May. However, he and Johnny Geldenhuys never worked well together and in early March he was fired. About the same time we were joined by two more men, Jack Pickering and Bill Burden. Towards the end of February much of the preparatory work had been completed and I was getting restless through not having enough work to do. Mr. Crawhall made a visit to the site about this time and I asked him if I could learn the job of a diamond-driller. He was not in favour of this but I was pleased a few weeks later when Johnny seconded me to Hennie Jansen to learn how to use the wagon-drill. This had its unpleasant aspects as for most of the time while drilling one was covered with a fine spray of water. However, this did not last long as my big chance came a few weeks later when three of the men decided to resign. This meant that the contract was threatened by a shortage of diamond-drillers and so I went to see Mr. Henderson, managing director of the Rhodesia office, and told him somewhat recklessly that I too would resign unless I could be more use and learn how to operate one of the diamond drills. Amazingly this worked and I was then given control of a drilling machine with instructions to call on Johnny whenever I felt I needed help.

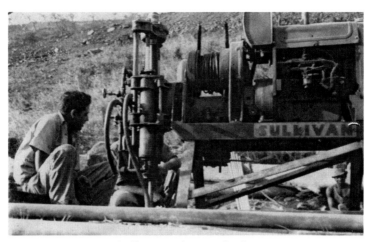

At my drilling machine. Rhodesia 1950

The holes were drilled by a machine comprising a large engine that drove a rotating head to which rods were fitted. A diamond bit mounted in tungsten carbide was attached to the end of the first rod so that when the engine rotated a hole was drilled in the rock. Rods came in 10 foot lengths and when one had passed through the head to its full length another would be added. For this work each machine was allocated the help of an African. Hardness of the rock layers varied and the skill lay in adjusting the speed of the machine to the quality of the rock through which one was drilling. The diamond bits were expensive and were worn out quickly if you tried to force the drilling through hard rock. So with experience you became attuned to the note of the engine. This gave an indication of the quality of rock being encountered and by making appropriate adjustments you could get more "footage" from each bit. I soon came to enjoy the work and had the added satisfaction of feeling that I was making a proper contribution to the project. Once the holes had been drilled to the requisite depth the pump man connected the top of the hole to the hose from his machine and liquid cement was pumped in under pressure.

We worked long hours during the day and ate together in the evening. Johnny and his wife, who everyone called the Missus, lived separately from the men but would occasionally join us for an evening meal. She was a delightful person and a calming influence on what was otherwise a fairly rough and coarse environment. After the first three months we exchanged our tented accommodation for individual small wooden "shacks" which sometimes had to be shared. I became good friends with a tough young man, Eddie Harding, who had come down from the 'Copper Belt' in Northern Rhodesia. During the weekends a lot of poker was played, usually accompanied by heavy drinking. I learned to play poker the hard way and lost heavily during the first few months, which resulted in having to sell the motorbike to cover my debts. Occasionally some of the Clifford Harris men came over to our mess to drink and play cards and there were one or two memorable fights in which Eddie was involved and one in which one of his drunken friends came after me with a carving knife.

The other form of recreation was to go to Salisbury – now Harare - if we had a free day over the weekend. This was usually accomplished either by hitchhiking or getting on a goods train when it stopped at the local siding. I was fortunate in that two of my cousins, Fay and Josephine, were living in Salisbury and I would sometimes stay the night with them. They were both young and attractive and the men would encourage me to ask them to join us but their enthusiasm was not reciprocated. The usual entertainment was going to the cinema or having a good meal in one of the cheap restaurants, inevitably accompanied by too much drinking on the part of the men. I also learned to drink brandy, which was the favourite tipple, but not to excess. I did, however, start smoking. Cigarettes were very cheap as Rhodesia was a major tobacco-producing country and those made from the floor sweepings, which were meant for the African population but smoked by many whites, cost one penny for a packet of eight. These packets carried delightful names such as "Tip Top", "Zig Zag" and "Top Hat".

My mother, who was a wonderful letter writer, kept in regular correspondence. She used to write a six- page letter every Sunday evening and this usually arrived on Thursday. I replied, albeit with a shorter letter, every seven to ten days. Sometime in May she told me that she had received a letter from Mr. Pateman, my previous headmaster, informing her that he had been able to reserve a place for me at St John's College Cambridge in October 1951 to read engineering. I felt, however, that I would prefer to take my BSc at 'Wits' before going up to Cambridge and after further correspondence between Pateman and the Tutor of Engineering at St John's, nothing further came of this.

In July, after I had been working on a diamond drill for three months my basic pay was increased from £2 to £7 per month. This followed a remark by Mr Henderson that he believed in paying a man what he was worth. This riled me somewhat as I was doing the same job as the man next to me who was getting £30 per month more. I asked him to bring the question of my pay to the attention of Mr. Crawhall when he visited the site later that month, but as this was not referred to again during the weeks that followed I unwisely gave Mr. Henderson an ultimatum that unless I got learner-driller's wages by the end of the month I would quit. He was not pleased and said he would write to Crawhall. I then received a scathing letter from Mr. Crawhall, pointing out that I had been given work experience through his good will and warning me of the dangers of seeking undue monetary reward at such an early stage of my career. He ended by saying that if I persisted in my attitude he would release me immediately but that I would have to repay the deposit made by the Company for my entry into Rhodesia. This of course I could not do and in any case by then I was feeling guilty for having behaved in such a foolish way, and so there was nothing for it but to climb down and apologise for what I had done. However, I must have eventually restored something of my reputation because after returning home at the end of the year I received a nice letter from Mr. Crawhall in which he wrote:

"I am pleased to tell you that Mr. Henderson has recommended that you be given a bonus cheque for £15 at the conclusion of your stay at Hunyani Poort.

It is with much satisfaction that I hear of your sound work and trust that what you have learnt on that contract will stand you in good stead in your future career."

Despite this unfortunate incident Johnny Geldenhuys continued to be very good to me. Pressure on the contract was building up and I began to work an extra shift on Sundays. Then in September Bill Ferriera left, which meant that I was the only diamond driller left on the job until further recruits arrived. For a period of time I also took over pumping the cement into the holes that had been drilled as we were left without a 'Pump Man' when Sarel De Beer departed. Our work was becoming urgent as treatment of the core trench leading to the spillway alongside the dam wall had to be completed before concrete could be laid in the latter. For a short period we were working 12 hours a day with half an hour off for lunch, but as I wrote to my mother, I was sure the hard work was doing me good and that the year was being of inestimable value to me. I could further reassure her that I was very fit with a tremendous appetite and putting on weight. By October we were out of the core trench and back to a normal timetable. I also became more solvent as I had received some bonus pay in lieu of the overtime worked and then in November a new bonus scheme was introduced depending on footage drilled and the number of expensive bits one had used to achieve this. I later broke the record by getting 139 feet drilled out of a single bit!

The end of the year was clouded by news that my mother was not well and had been admitted to hospital in Pietermaritzburg for tests for amoebic dysentery. This caused her to miss Elizabeth's 21st birthday party but happily she soon recovered her good health and returned to Johannesburg. The last few weeks at Hunyani were happy ones. Our main work had been completed although there was still quite a lot of tidying up to do. On the other hand Clifford Harris was in a race against time to complete the concreting of the spillway as the water level rose up the dam. There had been unexpectedly heavy rains and this was accomplished just in time. When the time came for my return home I was able to say a thankful and grateful farewell to Johnny and the Missus. They had been extraordinarily good to me throughout the year and I only appreciated later the burden of responsibility that Johnny must have felt in having me under his care. Henderson also came up trumps by paying my rail fare back to South Africa. And on the journey back I remember thinking how much I had learned and matured since leaving Johannesburg on the back of the truck eleven months earlier.

I returned home from Rhodesia the week before Christmas. It was a great joy being reunited with my mother and sister and to be living in comfortable and familiar surroundings. Elizabeth and I didn't have long together as, having spent the previous three years at home getting a BA at Wits, she decided to spread her wings and go to Cape Town University where she had signed up for a two year course in Social Sciences. After a happy family Christmas at home, I had a brief holiday in Durban with my cousin Corinne and then prepared to start University. At this time the accommodation at 17 Loch Avenue was rearranged. My mother, being hard up, decided to augment her income by having paying guests, or PGs as we called them. These were usually two young students of the same sex who shared the double room at the end of the house and who were treated very much as family, taking their breakfast and dinner with us. My mother charged them very little and I doubt this was of much economic benefit to her. However, as a result of their presence, I moved into the small workshop in the garden, which had been built for me when I was growing up. This was able to accommodate a bed, a desk and a chair and gave me a degree of independence that I much appreciated.

Just before starting at Wits I received a letter from the Secretary of the Transvaal Chamber of Mines confirming that I had been awarded a scholarship to study for the BSc Engineering (Civil) degree. The amount was £112 for 1951, to be paid in four quarterly payments, with tuition fees paid direct to the University by the Chamber of Mines. I was to be responsible for the £1 registration fee and any "deposits for breakages". This was very welcome and came as a surprise as I had given up hope of getting the scholarship after a difficult interview in which I seemed to be completely at cross purposes with those interviewing me.

On the strength of this and with what I had saved during my time in Rhodesia I bought my first car, the first in a long love affair with cars that has lasted throughout my lifetime. This was a small 1936 Morris 8 convertible for which I paid £100. I knew my mother would be very much against my owning a car at such a young age and so I left it at a friend's house before telling her what I had done. She was understandably annoyed and I responded by saying that I would do anything she wished providing I could retain it. She immediately said: "Well then Terence, I want you to stop smoking cigarettes", to which I could only agree. And so it is that I owe that little car a lot more than the pleasure it gave me, as I gave up cigarettes and turned to a pipe which I enjoyed for the next 25 years.

The first year at Wits was a restless one and I missed the freedom and rough life that I had experienced in Rhodesia. Our home in Parktown was within easy access of the University and I found interest in being able to mix with different social and racial groups. Wits had a strong liberal tradition and the worst of the Apartheid laws had not yet reached the statute book. So for the first time we white students were able to mix freely and on an equal basis with black and Indian South Africans, thereby widening our political horizons. Amongst the other students the engineers were regarded as a rather coarse and rowdy group, interested mainly in sport and without much political engagement whereas the medics were seen as the social and intellectual elite who dominated most of the liberal student organisations. Later, when I was studying medicine at the University of London, the reverse seemed to be largely the case.

For the first year all engineering students followed the same course that included Maths, Applied Maths, Physics and Chemistry. One of my clearest memories of this time is the maths lectures delivered to over 300 students in the Great Hall by a Mr. Olivier. He was a brilliant lecturer and used to cover the large blackboards with equations as he explained them to us. He was also a stern disciplinarian and seemed to have eyes in the back of his head so that anyone misbehaving or not paying attention would be greeted with a loud "Out, get out" and the miscreant would have to leave. For the most part it became a relaxed and carefree existence, attending most of the lectures but not doing much additional studying. There was a lot of time for socialising, with tennis, swimming and sport high on the agenda and I acquired a girlfriend, Pam Levene, with whose family I went on holiday to the South Coast of Natal in July. Later I somehow found myself in the University Boxing Team, fighting as a middleweight. I don't recall how this came about but perhaps it was because of the brawls in which I had been involved in Rhodesia. In any event, my boxing career came to an ignominious end when, during the match against Pretoria University which was held in the Johannesburg City Hall, I was knocked out in the first round.

One of the new friends I made was Sam Campbell. He was a few years older than most of us and an excellent mechanic, and was using this to help put himself through university. He lived at Rose Deep mine outside Johannesburg and I got into the habit of helping him repair cars in the workshop at his home over the weekends. Sometimes we would work through much of the night and I learned a lot from him. During a short vacation in early October, we drove to Cape Town in his Chevrolet van, he to see his girlfriend and me to visit Elizabeth. We had an enjoyable few days but on the way back, with Sam driving too fast, we skidded on the gravel surface and turned over. Neither of us was hurt but the car was damaged and we were stranded at a desolate spot 300 miles from Cape Town and 600 miles from Johannesburg. We hitchhiked to Sam's home, borrowed a Ford Truck from a friend of his and drove straight back to the scene of the accident. By this time I was ready for some sleep but Sam insisted that we hitch up the Chevrolet and tow it straight back to Jo'burg, sharing the driving as we went. Later in the year, and with Sam's advice, I sold the Morris and bought a 1936 Terraplane, known thereafter as "Black Fanny", which served me well on my many travels during the next three years.

As the end of the year approached, and with exams looming, I became aware of the need for more study if I was to pass. So at every opportunity I locked myself in my room in the garden and worked hard to prepare for them and by the time they arrived I was reasonably confident that I had passed. I had already decided that once they were over I would try and spend the long summer vacation, most of December and into early February, earning money as a diamond driller in Rhodesia. Cementation had nothing to offer but I was fortunate to be taken on by a firm with the delightful name of Squirrel and Popplewell, who had a drilling contract at the Rhodesian Iron and Steel Commission (RISCOM) at QueQue. So at the beginning of December Elizabeth and I set off in Black Fanny and drove to Rhodesia, she to spend two weeks with Fay and other friends in Salisbury and me to work at RISCOM. Unlike the previous year, we covered the distance without mishap and in two days rather than five. Elizabeth and I had always been close and now that we were in early adulthood the bonds became closer and we delighted in being together.

On arrival I met the foreman, a Mr. Stowe, who I was told drank heavily but was well liked and a good boss. I was also surprised to meet Hennie Jansen who had transferred to QueQue from Hunyani, and now had a young wife with a three-week old baby. I was soon at work, assisting one of the other drillers with the promise that I would be given my own machine in a few weeks. The hours were long, 6.30am to 6pm with an hour off for lunch, but there was a pleasant social club on the site and I was given a small rondavel (thatched hut) to myself. A little later I was hugely relieved to receive a telegram from my mother: "Successful. Passed in all your subjects. Simply splendid. Brilliant. Love Mum".

I spent Christmas with Fay and her friends in Mazoe, the first I had ever spent away from my mother, who went to "Montrose" with Elizabeth. On the way back I called in at Hunyani to see Johnny and the Missus but broke a spring getting there and had to leave the car with them. I then got a goods train back to QueQue that took nine hours to cover the 150 miles.

By the time New Year came I was thoroughly enjoying my life at RISCOM. It was a huge change from Varsity life and I enjoyed having time to myself to read and be more reflective. It was at this time that I began to think about changing my course from Civil to Mining Engineering, with a strong urge to follow in my father's footsteps. I had also become interested in the remarkable early history of the diamond and gold mining industries in South Africa with which Great Uncle Fred had been so intimately and profitably involved. In addition, I had made many good friends amongst the mining students during our combined first year studies. I felt there would be no difficulty in transferring my scholarship which, coming from the Chamber of Mines, I anticipated would be welcomed, and resolved to tell my mother of this decision when I returned home.

I had also become good friends with a young man named Colvin Leonard. He had arrived from Northern Rhodesia (Zambia) where he had grown up and where amongst other achievements he was holder of a Rhodesian and East African amateur boxing title. The mess at RISCOM was a popular place to congregate and it was there one evening that I embarked on a risky bet. A lot of publicity both on the radio and in the newspapers was being given to a world title fight between a boxer from South Africa, Vic Toweel, and an Irishman, Peter Keenan. One of the men in the mess, Paddy Casey, kept on talking about how Keenan was going to thrash Toweel. I got tired of this and one night rashly said that I would bet my Terraplane against his equally ancient Ford that Toweel would win. Paddy looked a bit uncertain but in view of all that he had said could not withdraw and the bet was sealed. Word got around as to what had happened so on the night of the big fight a large crowd gathered around the radio to listen to it live. Great was my relief when at the end of the 15 rounds Toweel was announced the winner. I then went over to Paddy and asked for the keys of his car, which he parted with somewhat reluctantly. The next morning was a Sunday and Colvin and I decided to celebrate by taking two girls we knew for a picnic at a farm nearby, and we proudly set off in my new acquisition. Alas, on the way back I got into a bad skid on the gravel surface and we left the road, crashed through some trees, and turned over. Fortunately no one was hurt, and with help from passers by we managed to right the car and get it back on the road. It seemed to be mechanically sound and so we set off home. However, what we had not thought of was that the water had drained from the radiator while the car was upside down. So just before we reached our destination the engine seized up, whereupon I returned the keys to Paddy.

Another more serious life-threatening event occurred some weeks later shortly before my return home. I had made my last weekend visit to Salisbury during which there had been heavy rains throughout the country and on the way back many of the rivers were in flood. In those days most of the bridges were low concrete causeways with a set of steel rails on each side about a foot above the level of the concrete. When the rivers flooded the water simply flowed over the causeway and the custom was for travellers to wait until the waters subsided sufficiently to allow a crossing. On my return journey I was held up by no fewer than four flooded bridges and at one of these I had to sleep in the car and then wait another twelve hours before I could cross. On this occasion there were a large number of cars on each side of the riverbank with occupants chatting and picnicking together. I joined some young men swimming in the river and then decided to make my way across the causeway and dive off the rail along its edge. The river was fast flowing and the water came nearly up to my waist. When I got to the middle of the bridge I eased my foot slowly forward, feeling for the rail to stand upon. However, it got sucked between the rail and the edge of the bridge and at the same time the force of the water knocked me forward so that my foot became trapped. Two of the men on the bank saw what had happened and tried to make their way to where I was but were swept off the bridge before they could reach me. I struggled on and eventually with a huge effort managed to pull myself up on the rail far enough to dislodge my foot and then floated exhausted down the river. By evening the river had gone down sufficiently to allow us to cross, and the foreman showed remarkable understanding when I told him why I was 36 hours late for work.

At the end of February I returned home. My mother agreed only reluctantly with my decision to change to mining engineering but permission was forthcoming from the University and the Chamber of Mines. One of the exciting things that happened during this year was that a few of us from the second year were allowed to join a tour of the mines in Southern Rhodesia, Northern Rhodesia and the Belgian Congo, spending two weeks in each country. This had been arranged for the third and final year students and travel was to be by road through Southern Rhodesia and then by rail in our own dedicated coach through the other two countries. I managed to persuade our lecturer, Mr. Ted Edwards, that we would not be a burden on the transport arrangements if I could take four of us in my car. He had seen the Terraplane about the campus and had doubts as to whether it would survive the trip but having told him of my previous experience with it in Rhodesia he finally agreed. So at the end of June we all set off on what turned out to be a most memorable trip, memorable not only for all the different mines we saw but also for the hospitality we encountered along the way. In Southern Rhodesia alone we were taken round six different properties, mining different metals and in widely different parts of the country. For the most part we slept out or in rough accommodation but we also enjoyed socialising at the various mine clubs where we were treated to barbecues, beer and sometimes dancing. On one occasion we even put out a rugby team but got soundly beaten by the locals. I took the opportunity of revisiting RISCOM when we passed through QueQue and was shattered to be told that Colvin Leonard had shot himself two months earlier. No reason could be given and I was deeply affected by this tragic waste of a young life. On reflection I could see no hint of trouble looming during the time that we had been good friends.

On the last section of the road trip in Rhodesia, whilst driving Black Fanny rather fast, the water pump housing tore loose from the cylinder block and went through the radiator. Alas, having performed perfectly until then, she now had to be towed to Bulawayo. There I was able to buy a second-hand radiator that I left to be fitted, after which she was stored with the other cars while we did the next part of the trip by rail. We went first to Wankie Colliery and then had two days luxuriating at the Victoria Falls Hotel where we spent time exploring the Falls and taking a trip up river to Kandahar Island. This all came back to me 46 years later during my 4x4 drive from London to Cape Town, when I had the experience of bungee-jumping off the famous Victoria Falls railway bridge, something I thought at the time I should have done rather earlier in my life!

From the Victoria Falls we crossed into Northern Rhodesia and visited the large lead and zinc mine at Broken Hill where we again played rugby against the mine team and again were beaten. Our next few visits were to the mines on the Copper Belt in the northern part of the country. Here we were impressed by the modern mechanical methods of mining, which were every bit as advanced as those on the Witwatersrand. Again hospitality was outstanding and in our free time we played golf and also managed a draw against the Mufulira girls hockey team. From there our railway coach was taken by a wood-burning steam engine to Elizabethville in the Belgian Congo. The sight of the sparks emitting from the funnel of the engine at night was very dramatic and the bush had to be cleared for a quarter of a mile on each side of the tracks so that fires were not started. We spent much of the next ten days visiting the huge open cast mines run by the Union Minière du Haut Katanga and enjoying the European-style culture of the Congo where initially it was a surprise to hear many of the blacks speaking French. This all came to a sudden and disastrous end a few years later when the Belgians were driven out by the murderous Mobuto. When our time in the Congo came to an end we retraced our steps by rail to Bulawayo where we collected the cars and drove home without further event. It had been a hugely enjoyable and worthwhile experience.

The rest of the year passed tamely in comparison and by the time exams came I knew I had not done enough work to be sure of passing. I decided, however, to again make use of my knowledge of diamond drilling to earn some money during the long Christmas vacation. I approached Squirrel and Popplewell and they offered me a short contract drilling for copper in Northern Rhodesia. So back there I went six months after my previous visit. This time I decided to hitchhike, which turned out to be a more ambitious challenge than I had imagined. I left Johannesburg with a small rucksack, having sent on a trunk with my necessary clothes and belongings by rail to Kitwe, which was the main town on the Copper Belt. The journey started well with a lift by friends of the family all the way to Salisbury. However, the next day I had difficulty getting out of town and then had a series of short lifts to a remote part of the country where I was dropped off just before noon. There I waited until early evening by which time I was getting desperate when a young Afrikaans farmer and his wife stopped, took pity on me and kindly put me up for the night. The next morning after breakfast I was given sandwiches for the road and deposited at the spot where they had picked me up the previous evening. My luck now changed and after waiting a short time I was picked up by a splendid man who introduced himself as Vice Admiral Sir Anthony Morse. He was a great conversationalist and used to get so carried away with what he was saying that I occasionally had to remind him that he had an extra gear to change into. En route to Lusaka, where he dropped me off, we drove through the wild scenery of the Zambesi valley. Much of this area was flooded after the huge Kariba dam was built across the Zambesi river five years later. The next day I got a lift with three young men who drove dangerously fast but who got me safely to Broken Hill. There I spent the night at the Great Northern Hotel, run by a Mrs M English, and which was quite the worst hotel I had ever stayed in. The next morning I left early with an elderly gentleman who had three whiskies for breakfast at a pub along the road and was surprised that I didn't follow suit. He dropped me at Ndola and then it was two easy lifts to my destination at Kitwe. There I met Mr. Squirrel of Squirrel and Popplewell who drove me the next day to a camp in the bush about 20 miles distant from Kitwe where the firm was drilling for copper. With my arrival there were now five in the camp; a young Afrikaner Johan Taljard, his wife, mother-in-law and sister-in-law. I took over from someone who had left unexpectedly and after a few days with Johan, he and I worked alternate twelve hour shifts, from six to six. The camp was crude but comfortable and the women provided good meals, with Grace said beforehand in Afrikaans. The mother-in-law, Mrs. Bezuidenhout, took quite a shine to me and I recall one evening when she had had too much brandy I spent an embarrassing time fending off her advances. I loved the night shifts. The drilling rig was well lit and although the bush was in darkness, all sorts of interesting noises would come from it. Large moths were attracted by the light. These would be eaten by raucous toads, some of whom would then be eaten by snakes. I had two Africans to help me but could not communicate with them beyond what the work involved. However, I never recall feeling lonely and enjoyed the adventure of this new experience. Unfortunately it came to a premature end as towards the end of December I heard from my mother that, having passed in the four major subjects of Geology, Mining, Physics and Mechanical Engineering, I had failed in two subjects (Civil and Fuels) and would have to write supplementary exams in these before being allowed to proceed to the third year. So at the end of January I returned by rail to Johannesburg and fortunately passed both examinations. Thereafter I took a more responsible attitude towards my studies and had no further problems with examinations. Thankfully my scholarship was not affected.

My mother had an amazing capacity for friendship and we had a stream of visitors to our home at 17 Loch Avenue. I also had the pleasure of Elizabeth's company as having completed her BA in Social Science in Cape Town she returned to Johannesburg at the end of 1952 and was now living at home and working for the Mental Health Society. Our age difference of three years had become less noticeable and we shared many friends. She had always been a good pianist and I delighted in listening to her, sometimes being able to judge her mood by the way she played. My mother, who also played the piano but not as well as Elizabeth, had instilled in me a love of music and one of our extravagances was to attend concerts given by the Johannesburg City Orchestra or by visiting musicians from abroad. There were also excellent plays and musicals and I remember enjoying "Oklahoma" and "Annie Get Your Gun".

During the third year we continued to have a substantial practical component to our course. Apart from experience in the deep gold mines of the Rand, which spread for a distance of 30 miles to the East and West of Johannesburg, we had two further mining tours. The first was in April when we visited some of the Base Metal mines of the Eastern Transvaal. On this occasion we were accompanied by Mr Percy Crewell, senior lecturer in the department, and again we travelled by car, camping out at many places along the way unless our hosts allowed us to sleep in vacant mine sheds or similar rough accommodation. We started the tour at the huge open cast iron ore mine at Thabazimbi, and then went on to two separate tin mines at Zaaiplaats and Rooiberg before spending a few days at the picturesque village of Pilgrims Rest. This had been the centre of a gold rush to the Barberton area in the 1870's, before gold was discovered on the Witwatersrand. The village was largely preserved as it had been during the rush, with an excellent small museum that gave a vivid insight into the history of those turbulent times. Finally we went to the large asbestos mine at Havelock, which was just inside the Swaziland border.

In May we had a short tour of the Kimberley diamond mines, where we saw the famous 'Big Hole'. This had been excavated by hand in the 1870's to bring the diamondiferous 'blue ground' to the surface for sorting. When this hole became too deep to continue mining from the surface, shafts were sunk alongside the pipe and the ground retrieved by regular mining methods. This was a fascinating visit for me as Great Uncle Fred had been intimately involved in the diamond fields in the early days. As a relatively young man he had the good fortune to be farming near Colesberg 'kopje' (hillock), which was the first diamond pipe to be discovered in 1871 and which later became Kimberley Mine. Prior to this, in 1867, a large diamond had been found on the banks of the Orange River and soon several thousand prospectors were scouring the river banks for alluvial diamonds. However, their source remained unknown until the discovery of five diamondiferous 'pipes' near Kimberley, of which Colesberg 'kopje' was one of the richest. News of the discovery prompted a huge rush of diggers and prospectors and by the end of the year there were over 50,000 men in the area. Amongst them was Fred who, having quit his farm, was amongst the first to acquire valuable claims where the pipe outcropped. Soon many small mining companies had been formed and I believe that for a while he was associated in one of these with Cecil Rhodes. The latter had arrived in Kimberley towards the end of 1871, having travelled by ox-wagon from Natal where he had been sent for the sake of his health and where he had been trying unsuccessfully to grow cotton. Rhodes soon realised the need to consolidate the industry both for technical reasons as the mines became deeper and for creating a monopoly with respect to the production and marketing of diamonds. He was a shrewd speculator and by 1880 he and a few others were able to form the De Beers Mining Company that had strong holdings throughout the diamond fields. His main competitor was Barney Barnato who had arrived from the East End of London in 1873 and who had gained control of Kimberley Central Mines. Rhodes set about acquiring the latter and after several failures he was eventually successful and De Beers Consolidated Mines Ltd was formed in 1888. While in Kimberley we visited the Kimberley Club and I saw there a framed copy of the cheque for £5,338,650, which Rhodes had paid for the purchase of Kimberley Central. Another part of the deal was that Barnato was given membership of the Club, Jews having been excluded until that time.

After having made a small fortune in Kimberley, Great Uncle Fred went to the Witwatersrand when gold was discovered there in 1886. He arrived after much of the ground surrounding the outcrops had been staked, but he shrewdly judged that the reef would continue in depth and so acquired land further out, calculated on the incline of the reef at the surface. This proved to be correct and so he became known as "Deep Level English" amongst the mining community on the Rand. Having added to his fortune he retired to England in the mid-1890's where he bought, and lavishly restored, Addington Palace near Croydon, which had previously been the country home of the Archbishops of Canterbury. I mention this brief history because our family owes so much to him. He and his wife Kitty (neé Devenish), who was the eldest of thirteen, had no children of their own and before Fred died in 1909 he established the F.A. English Will Trust, a small portion of which came to our family. This eventually paid for my school education and also provided me with an inheritance of £2,000 when I reached the age of 21.

It was towards the end of this year, after having received notification of this inheritance that a new star appeared on my horizon and I began to think about the possibility of switching to medicine. I was enjoying my studies at Wits but simply thought I might be a better doctor than an engineer. I had also come to know and be influenced by my mother's youngest brother, Max Lund, who had qualified in medicine at Edinburgh and was now amongst the first surgical specialists practising in Natal. He had become for me somewhat of a father figure and I admired him immensely so I discussed the matter with him and was pleased by his encouraging response. Having decided to change careers I decided to change countries. My initial thought was to go to Edinburgh but Max suggested London would be a better option and that Guy's was an excellent medical school with a strong tradition of welcoming South African students. When I approached my

Professor and one of the senior lecturers in the department they proved to be surprisingly sympathetic and with their strong recommendations I put in an application to Guy's Hospital Medical School. Great was my joy when the Dean's reply came back that he would be prepared to accept me without interview providing I passed my BSc Engineering degree, which I had intended to complete anyway. My mother and Elizabeth were both delighted by my decision to do medicine and we had a very happy Christmas at 17 Loch Avenue, accompanied by Aunt Doreen and cousins Corinne and Josephine.

My last year at Wits passed happily and smoothly except for a serious event towards the end of the year that nearly upset my plans to do medicine. Before that however, during the vacation month of July, two of my friends, Paul Mortimer and Bob Bovell and I had managed to secure paid employment to run a geological survey at an asbestos mine in a desolate part of the Karroo near the small village of Prieska. We set off with an official from the head office in Johannesburg. On the way his car broke down but fortunately I was able to fix it. When we arrived at the mine, he was greeted with the Mill Manager's resignation. So because of my perceived mechanical skills I was appointed temporary Mill Manager with a nice small office of my own in the Mill, while Paul and Bob had to sweat it out in the sun all day running the survey. However, we all enjoyed our time there except for an incident that occurred shortly before our departure. I had brought a rifle with me and soon after arrival we visited the local farmer and asked if we could shoot on his land. He agreed to this but requested that we confine ourselves to rabbits and not anything larger. When the day came that we were finally able to go shooting we had been out a long time without luck when, after stalking a 'dassie' (rock-rabbit), I suddenly saw a male springbok at some distance and without hesitating to think fired and killed it. However, the thrill of the hunt soon disappeared when I examined the buck. First of all it was so beautiful that I determined I would never again kill an animal for sport. And then to my horror I saw that the point of both of its horns had been sawn off suggesting that it had previously been captured, if not domesticated. There was nothing for it but to take the buck to the farmer's homestead and explain what had happened. Mr. Vlok was not in and his wife, who looked very grave when she heard my story, suggested that we return at noon the next day which was a Sunday. I decided to return alone and was met by Mr. Vlok on his 'stoep' (veranda). He asked his wife to bring

41

coffee and then having reminded me of his generosity for allowing us to shoot on his land, berated me for not having obeyed his instructions. He went on to tell me how he was in the process of restocking his farm with springbok and that he had caught the one I had shot in the Kalahari. It was a young animal at the time and he had fallen off his horse in the process, injuring his shoulders. The buck had then been kept for a short while in an enclosure near the house before being released to the wilds of his farm. I was absolutely mortified. There were further recriminations about how could I as an educated English-speaking South African have done such a thing to a poor Afrikaans sheep-farmer. All I could do was to apologise profusely and having had my offer of payment refused I returned to the mine feeling absolutely wretched. After returning home I wrote him a letter in Afrikaans again apologising for what I had done and seeking his forgiveness. And there the shameful matter ended.

The other foolish event I was involved in, which nearly had much more serious consequences, occurred at the end of the academic year just before our final examinations. After having enjoyed a splendid Final Year Dinner at the Wanderer's Club, and having had rather too much to drink, someone suggested that we should mount a 'Panty Raid' on the Women's Residence. This was something that was happening in American Universities at the time but not yet in South Africa. So twelve of us drove to the Residence and, having entered the grounds, three of us managed to climb a drainpipe and get into a girl's room. I sat on the windowsill while my friends asked the two startled girls for underwear to throw to the rest of our group waiting below. At this point the Dean of the Residence stormed in and chased the three of us back down the drainpipe, after which we got into our cars and drove off. What we hadn't realised was that one of the two who had entered the room had dropped a signed menu card on the floor with all our names on it. So the next day we were called before the Principal of the University and told that the Dean, who took the gravest view of what had happened, had declared that she would resign unless those who had entered the girls room were sent down for a year. The three of us owned up and then spent a very uncomfortable week not knowing whether we would be able to sit our exams and during which I could see my plans for doing medicine coming to an abrupt end or at best being delayed for a year. However, we went to see the Dean of Engineering, Professor G R Bozzoli, or 'Boz', as he was known to everyone at Wits. He was stern but sufficiently sympathetic so that after interceding on our behalf with Principal Raikes we were allowed to sit our exams and graduate. We heard later that the Dean did in fact resign.

So the year eventually ended well. In retrospect I do not regret the four years studying engineering. I think this helped to engender a logical problem-solving mind and to the extent I have developed this, it has served me well in my life as a surgeon. Before leaving for England I paid a visit to Uncle Fred who, like my father and his younger brother Henry, had fought throughout the First World War, and who during the Somme had been one of the few survivors of the Battle of Delville Wood where the South African brigade had fought so valiantly in July 1916. Fred had married late and he and his wife, Hawkie,

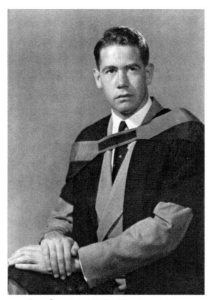

Graduation, BSc. Engineering, Witwatersrand University. 1954

lived in peace and isolation on the banks of the river Krom in the Eastern Cape. Indeed I had to open and close twelve gates on the road between the nearest village and the modest house that he himself had built. I had previously felt that Fred had admired my father so much that I never quite measured up to his expectations. However, this visit was a warm and happy one. I think he was touched that I had come to see him before I departed South Africa and when I was leaving he took off the signet ring that he had inherited from his namesake, Great Uncle Fred, and gave it to me. This remains one of my most treasured possessions, having been made from some of the first gold to be mined on the Rand, and with the inscription "From W.G.B. 1889" on its undersurface. I don't know who "W.G.B." was but presume he was one of Great Uncle Fred's friends or associates during his early days in Johannesburg. When each of my sons, Arthur and William, reached 21 I gave them exact replicas of the ring, which I continue to wear.

I had booked a passage on the Carnarvon Castle, one of the Union Castle Mailboats, due to leave Cape Town on 24th December arriving Southampton on 6th January, so was able to attend my graduation ceremony before departure. My mother had sold 17 Loch Avenue earlier in the year since when we had been living in a flat in Rosebank. Elizabeth had received an offer from Dr Maxwell Jones, a friend of Uncle Max's from Edinburgh days, who was head of the psychiatric hospital at Belmont in Surrey and she was due to follow me to England in two weeks. So a few days before Christmas I took the train to Cape Town and having said goodbye to various friends and relations boarded the Carnarvon Castle late afternoon on Christmas Eve. My cabin was at the rear of the ship and seemed to be just above the propellers. As we steamed out into the Cape rollers I began to feel distinctly queasy but I told myself that sea-sickness was largely psychological and proceeded to the dining room for our festive first meal. However, I had hardly finished reading the menu before reality set in and I had to hurry back to my cabin where I was violently ill for the next twelve hours. Thereafter we entered calmer waters and the voyage became a delightful experience. This was before the days of mass air travel and there were lots of young people on board with all sorts of activities arranged for our pleasure. As we drew closer to England the skies became darker and by the time we arrived we were in the depths of a bitter English winter. I was met at Waterloo by one of my ex-girlfriends, Ann Van Tilburg, who had kindly arranged for me to share accommodation in a flat in Walton Street, South Kensington, with another South African, Dennis Claude. He was working for a firm of architects in the City, and our Irish landlady, Miss McMahon, was an absolute treasure. The rent was £5 per week and rather romantically the lighting was all by gas as was the stove and heating via a small fire in the living room. We cooked for ourselves, a lot of porridge and pasta, as having been brought up in South Africa this was a skill we had not acquired, and Miss McMahon would occasionally take pity on us and bring us down a dish of her own making. Within the first week, and despite the wet and the snow and the cold, I knew I was going to like England.

Chapter 3
Canada and Medical School

Soon after arrival in London I reported to the Secretary of the Medical School at Guy's Hospital. He suggested that in view of my degree in Engineering I should be able to get exemption from two of the first year subjects, namely Physics and Chemistry. Furthermore that if I passed A-level Biology before October I would be able to start in the second year of the medical course. For this I would need to register with London University as an external student and then sign up with an appropriate College to read Biology. The A-level course would have started in October so I would have missed the first three months and the examination would be held in July.

I accepted his advice and within a fortnight had started a course in Biology at the University Tutorial College, a small private college in Bloomsbury. This I soon found utterly depressing. The small classrooms were crowded and cold, the lectures disappointing, and too much time seemed to be spent dissecting frogs and dogfish. Within a fortnight I had decided that there must be better ways of spending my time and that I would revert to my original plan of starting 1st MB at Guy's in October. Accordingly I began to look for a job. Elizabeth had arrived in England by now and was enjoying her work at Belmont Psychiatric Hospital in Surrey. Dr Maxwell Jones, for whom she was working, initially suggested there might be a job for me at the hospital but then changed his mind. I made use of the time to explore London and visit many of the tourist attractions such as the National Gallery, Madame Tussauds, the Festival Hall and the Tate where I particularly wanted to see Rodin's "The Kiss". I enjoyed the new experience of the English Pub, both posh ones around where we lived in South Kensington and the rougher 'musical' ones in the East End such as the "Prospect of Whitby" in Wapping. I also went to Addington Palace in

Croydon to see where Great Uncle Fred had lived and where my father and two of his sisters used to take their holidays while they were at school in England. Most of the beautiful grounds had been taken over by a golf club, and the large house that was now owned by Croydon County Council, had been leased to the Royal School of Church Music. While there, I visited St Mary's Church which is adjacent to the house and is where Great Uncle Fred and several other members of the family are buried and where, in due course, I would like to join them.

After a while, a new and brighter star appeared on the horizon. I began to realise that perhaps the best opportunity of getting a good job and supplementing my capital, rather than seeing it diminish, would be to use what I had been trained for and seek employment in mining exploration in Canada. I chose Canada for three reasons. I knew that as a country it had become aware of its vast potential mineral wealth and that accordingly there was a lot of activity in geological and geophysical exploration. I also knew that much of this was seasonal taking place predominantly during the summer, when the remoter areas were more accessible. And finally Canada had always appealed to me as a country to visit. So within a few weeks I had booked a passage on one of the oldest Cunarders, SS Franconia, and on 5th March set sail from Liverpool to Halifax. This was a very different voyage from the Cape Town to Southampton crossing of a few months earlier. The weather was dull and cold throughout and there was none of the fun and light-hearted activity we had enjoyed on the Carnarvon Castle. Many of the passengers were Irish immigrants and my cabin-mate was an ex GI who had married an English woman during the War and then spent the next decade trying to save enough money to get him and his family back to a milk-round in Chicago.

On arrival in Halifax I boarded the train that night for Toronto. The journey took 36 hours and much of the time we passed through forests covered in thick snow. When I got to Toronto I checked in at the YMCA and after getting a list of mining exploration companies from the telephone book I began knocking on doors, armed with a copy of my degree certificate. During the next two days I was interviewed by no fewer than sixteen firms and was rewarded by securing what sounded like two excellent jobs. The first was with Teck Exploration Company involving a geophysical prospect in the Yukon Territory which, however, was only due to commence in mid-May. The second was to start immediately and last two months, and was with Technical Mines Consultants Ltd. I was to go initially to a property in

Northern Quebec that was being investigated for copper. Having obtained an advance on my salary I bought a sleeping bag, boots, warm coat and a woolly hat with ear flaps to wear over a balaclava and then set off by train to Noranda accompanied by the Chief Geologist, Don James. From there we flew into the property that had been "staked" the previous autumn on the basis of an electromagnetic anomaly, picked up by an airborne geophysical survey. We landed on a frozen lake and I was handed a pair of snowshoes for the walk in deep snow to the nearby camp. It was bitterly cold, with temperatures ranging between +5º and 20º below zero, so before the pilot left with Don James I arranged that he would bring me some warm one-piece long underwear and heavy duty mittens on his next visit.

The camp comprised two wooden shacks. One was for the cook and his kitchen; the other for the four diamond-drillers, a handy man, and me. All the men were French Canadians and some expressed surprise when they learned I was from South Africa and not black. The day started at 5.45 am with a loud shout of "Roll Out" from the cook, followed by lunch at noon and supper at 6 pm. I got on well with the drillers, part of my time being spent studying and logging the core they retrieved and preparing samples from the mineralised zone to be sent away to assay for copper. The rest of the time I spent on my own on snowshoes completing a ground magnetometer survey over the rest of the property. I loved these days, deep in the snowbound woods, very quiet apart from an occasional birdcall and very far from civilisation. After a month, and with the work nearly completed, we made a rather hurried departure. Spring was on its way, the lake at Noranda was becoming unsafe for planes with skis to land on, and we were told that Head Office did not want us to remain in camp for the duration of the 'break-up' which might mean staying on for several more weeks.

As soon as I returned to Toronto I was dispatched to the booming uranium area at Blind River on the shores of Lake Huron in northeastern Ontario. The geologist Franc Joubin, who was head of Technical Mines Consultants, had been primarily responsible for discovering uranium in this area. He had received financial backing from Joseph Hirshorn, an immigrant from Latvia who, by 1960, when he sold the last of his uranium stock, had made over $100 million from his investments. (He later collected one of the world's largest private art collections of paintings and sculptures from the nineteenth and twentieth centuries, which he eventually donated to the Smithsonian Institute in Washington.) I was based at Lake Nordic

Uranium Mines where there was an active drilling programme but as yet no mine. I spent most of my time logging the core and testing it for radioactivity. The drilling results were kept a close secret as stocks and shares fluctuated wildly on Bay Street in Toronto as rumours of rich new finds circulated. Here I enjoyed a much more comfortable camp than the one in Northern Quebec and I revelled in the glorious spring weather after the cold winter months.

By mid-May it was time to return to Toronto and prepare for my next job in the Yukon. I found on arrival that Teck Exploration needed me a week later than originally planned so I asked them to give me the equivalent of my air fare to Whitehorse in order that I could buy a car and drive across Canada to Vancouver and then fly the shorter distance from there to Whitehorse. Happily they agreed and after two days studying the advertisements for cars I bought a 1951 Chevrolet coupé from a very pleasant couple Mr and Mrs Matheson. They befriended me and took me on a day's outing to Niagara Falls before I set off on my travels. At that time the trans-Canada highway had yet to be built so the first part of the journey was across gravel roads in northern Ontario. I picked up two young hitchhikers for company who were heading for Winnipeg, and each evening would drop them off at the local jail to seek accommodation, whilst I sought more comfortable lodgings. It took a full two days to drive across the flat wheat fields of Manitoba and Saskatchewan and then after traversing much of Alberta the scenery became more dramatic as I drove towards the Rocky Mountains. I left Banff in a flurry of snow but made a detour to Lake Louise when the sun came out leaving everything looking beautiful. Then across Kootenay Bay by ferry and on to Vancouver, completing the 3,200 miles in just six days. The Chevrolet had behaved well and I had no difficulty selling it for the same price I had paid in Toronto. After exploring Vancouver for a day I flew to Whitehorse where I received a message from Jim Walker, who was in charge of the project. He explained that he was delayed and that I should make my own way to Burwash Landing, 200 miles north of Whitehorse on the Alaska Highway and thence to our camp at Arch Creek, 35 miles west of the Highway. There I was to meet other members of the party. I left Whitehorse early on 28th May and after getting directions from Burwash Landing made my way to the Hudson Bay Company camp where I was given supper and then walked with my gear the last six miles to Arch Creek. It was an exhilarating feeling to be so alone, not entirely sure of the way, and with a sense of adventure which had been stimulated by reading Robert Service's poems "Songs of a Sourdough" while I was in Whitehorse. On arrival in camp I was met by Joe Jaquot the cook, two elderly prospectors, one of whom had walked into the Yukon as a young man during the Klondike gold rush of 1896 and had remained ever since, and an American, Frank Mills, with whom I was to work. There were also six Indians who had been hired on a temporary basis to cut lines through the woods for a grid on which the geophysical survey would be based. Joe was an interesting character being the son of a celebrated French pastry cook, who came to the Yukon to trade and married one of the local Indian women. He had developed a profitable hunting business - all land east of the Alaska Highway was open to hunting whereas that to the west, where we were, was protected ground – but needed to find extra employment outside the hunting season.

Frank and I soon became firm friends and there then began one of the happiest summers of my life. We were camped alongside a stream in the foothills of the Mt St Elias range and the scenery was magnificent. There was a saltlick on a hill near the camp to which mountain sheep made frequent visits. There were also grizzly bears in the vicinity and one day we came home to find Joe had shot one, but not before it had entered our camp. On another occasion a grizzly chased some of the Indians up a tree, after which they would not go out without a rifle. Frank and I spent all day on the geophysical survey. This involved much climbing up and down the mountains and I soon became extremely fit. We would always stop for lunch beside a stream, during which we would make a small fire for tea and then enjoy smoking our pipes before continuing with the work. We shared a small tent in which I had constructed a bed made out of spruce boughs that proved to be amazingly comfortable. As summer approached the days lengthened and we could sit outside our tent and read late into the evening. I had got into the habit of reading a lot during my time in Quebec and Ontario and arrived with a good stock of books. These included the abridged volume of Toynbee's "A Study of History" which I had bought in Vancouver; the Essays of Emerson and Montaigne; Walt Whitman's "Leaves of Grass"; the collected plays of Eugene O'Neil, and novels by Faulkner and John Dos Passos amongst others. Frank, who at one time had considered a career in journalism, was widely read and made an ideal companion. Despite living more or less on top of each other there was never any lack of harmony and I began to appreciate for the first time the nature of true friendship.

One of our luxuries was to spend an occasional weekend at Burwash Landing. This was on Mile1093 Alaska Highway, the latter having been built by the Americans during the Second World War to connect Edmonton in Alberta with Fairbanks in Alaska. It comprised a small hotel with a beer parlour, a filling station and garage, and an Indian settlement nearby. It was here that on one occasion I met Joe's mother, who must have weighed all of 350lbs but who declared that she still enjoyed riding whenever she could find a horse strong enough to support her. Burwash was one of the few places along the Highway where you could get fuel, food and accommodation. The hotel was owned by a lazy American married to a Finnish lady, and she in turn had brought out two charming Finnish girls to help with work in the hotel. Frank became friendly with Matta and I became fond of Vieno, so they soon became an added attraction for visiting Burwash. Vieno, at 36, was thirteen years older than me but the difference in age and background did not provide a barrier to our deepening affection for each other in the romantic circumstances in which we found ourselves. After I returned to England we kept in touch and then after a few years I heard she was back in Finland and about to be married.

Jim Walker had joined us in June in our attempts to identify a possible extension of the nickel orebody being mined by the Hudson Bay Mining Company six miles away. For this we employed geophysical techniques that depend on the physical properties of different rocks. For example nickel sulphide acts as a conductor if a current is passed through it, so by using a generator to transmit a current in the direction of a receiving coil, and then plotting the results on a grid with stations of known distance apart, abnormalities of conductivity can be identified. These can then be explored by drilling. By mid-July we had largely completed our work at Arch Creek with only a few isolated claims still to explore. As soon as this had been done we moved camp to Vulcan Creek, somewhat closer to Whitehorse but even more mountainous, so that it was difficult terrain to work on. Here more rocks were exposed so we could supplement the geophysical work with geological mapping. As autumn approached the trees turned a rich colour of gold and red, and winter was heralded by a heavy snowfall on the mountains in late August. It began to get colder and we needed to light a stove in our tent each night. We also had some wonderful viewings of the Aurora Borealis – or "Northern Lights" – which can be spectacular in this part of the world. The fieldwork finished slightly earlier than anticipated and after a final few days in Burwash we returned to Whitehorse where I had my beard shaved off before Frank and I flew to Edmonton. There we boarded the Canadian National Super Continental that took us in great style to Toronto. On the journey we spent many happy hours in the luxurious Viewing Dome, drinking beer and watching the Canadian scenery slip by. Jim Walker had flown directly to Toronto where he completed the analysis of our geophysical surveys. This initially was not encouraging but on further exploration the following year an interesting conduction anomaly was detected which on drilling proved to be ore- bearing. This, however, was not of sufficient value to warrant mining in such distant parts where the costs are proportionately higher.

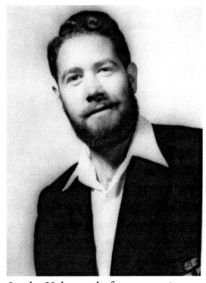

In the Yukon – before returning to England. September 1955.

Frank and I spent a few days together at the Walker House Hotel, which was his favourite 'watering-hole' in Toronto and then I set off by bus to New York where I boarded the 'Ile de France' on 24th September, arriving back in England just in time to start at Guy's on 1st October. By a strange coincidence, whilst boarding the ship in New York, I bumped into Brookes Parkman and her recently married husband, Cal Woodard. Brookes was from Boston and had stayed with us in Johannesburg for several weeks during 1952 when she accompanied Gwendoline Carter who was researching a book on current politics in South Africa, later published under the title "The Politics of Inequality". We had all become very fond of Brookes, who was a wonderfully attractive and intelligent person, and had kept in touch after her departure from South Africa. Cal was from North Carolina and had become a successful lawyer on Wall Street. However, like me, he had decided to change direction, and was en route to Pembroke College, Cambridge, where he had been accepted to read History, with the view of becoming an academic historian. We had lots of time during the voyage to talk about why we were changing careers and discuss some of the uncertainties that lay ahead. These conversations were continued when I used to visit Brookes and Cal in Cambridge while I was experiencing difficulty with carrying on with medicine. Cal successfully completed his degree and ended up as Professor of History of Law at the University of West Virginia in Charlottesville. Sadly Brookes died soon after their second child was born.

London was damp and grey when I returned. I had arranged to stay at London House in Bloomsbury, which was an establishment for male students from the Commonwealth. I began by sharing a room with two other South Africans but later managed to get a cubicle of my own. Having reported to Guy's I started on my 1st MB studies. Although, as mentioned, I had gained exemption from Physics and Chemistry, I decided it would be sensible to refresh my knowledge in these subjects, leaving Biology as the only examination to sit. This was a good decision, as although I didn't care for Chemistry, Biochemistry was interesting and the Physics lectures outstanding. We were a class of 80, amongst who were ten girls, and my fellow students, the great majority of whom had come straight from school, seemed to me very immature. I partially solved this problem by deciding to find companionship on the rugby field. During my last year at Wits I had on one occasion played for the University 1st XV and I was now very fit after my strenuous life in Canada. It was therefore with much pleasure that I was invited three weeks after arrival to go on a tour to the West Country with the Hospital 1st XV. The captain of the team was another South African, Stan Cooke, also from a Johannesburg mining background, and he and I became life-long friends, being godparents to each other's children. Three other members of the team were South Africans: Aubrey Buirski, 'Van' Van den Berg and Michael Russell, all of whom became good friends. I played a lot of rugby during that first year. Before the War Guy's had a very successful team and as a result retained a fixture list which included many strong clubs such as Cambridge, Blackheath, Wasps, Coventry and Bedford. We didn't win many of these matches though we did get to the Finals of the Inter- Hospitals Cup competition, but sadly were beaten for the second year running by St Mary's.

Elizabeth met me when I returned to London and soon thereafter she introduced me to Dave Auger whom she had met on the boat from South Africa at the beginning of the year. Dave was an engineer on the Union Castle line and they had been seeing a lot of each other whenever he was in port. I liked him and a few weeks later Elizabeth told me that they were to marry. Dave needed to serve another two years before he could get his Chief Engineer's ticket but would then leave the Merchant Navy. They seemed very happy with each other and I was able to reassure our mother that Elizabeth had found a man whom I believed was worthy of her.

At this time Mum was finalising her plans to spend a year on the island of Ibiza. This resulted from her friendship with Nancy Lister whom she had known since schooldays. Indeed Nancy's husband, Dr Hugh von Menghishausen, had delivered me into this world. Nancy, who was also a widow, was a fine artist and having decided to spend a year painting on Ibiza asked Mother to accompany her. They arrived on the island in November and Elizabeth and I were invited to join them for a few weeks over Christmas and the New Year. This we did, travelling first to Paris and then by train to Barcelona, where we took the overnight boat to Ibiza. This was an uncomfortable crossing as the Mediterranean was rough and, with many of the passengers being sick in the crowded quarters below deck, I preferred to spend the night in a chair on deck. Ibiza had yet to become a popular tourist destination and the only way of getting to the island was by weekly boats from either Barcelona or Valencia. It had great charm and everything was very cheap. Nancy and my mother had started in a small hotel and then moved to a set of rooms overlooking the harbour which they rented for 20 pesetas a day, which in English money at that time was worth about three shillings. Food was equally cheap and my mother was able to live comfortably on £15 per month. By the time Elizabeth and I arrived they had already got to know a number of the small but interesting "foreign colony" of writers and artists who lived on the island. Nancy was painting – she did portraits of both Elizabeth and me during our stay – and my mother was holding English 'conversations' with some of the local inhabitants. One of these was the man in charge of the prison. There was very little crime on Ibiza and one day he expressed his concerns that he might soon be out of a job as there was only one prisoner left in the goal. This man had been serving a long sentence but was soon to be discharged and his worry was that because he had to send a return to the office in Spain every month, he feared that if he had no prisoners it was likely he would be dismissed. My mother suggested that a possible solution might be to come to an arrangement with the departing prisoner whereby he would be free during the day but continue to use the goal to sleep in at night, at least until another prisoner was admitted, so that the appropriate returns might continue to be sent to the mainland. This was accepted as an excellent idea and the story soon got passed around amongst the jailer's friends, with much approval for the 'good sense' of the English lady.

Elizabeth and I had a most enjoyable three weeks on Ibiza. The weather was much warmer than mid-winter England; we met interesting people and explored other parts of what was a charming island. We were also able to have long discussions with our mother about what a momentous year it had been for both of us. She of course wanted to hear all about Dave from Elizabeth and Canada and Guy's from me, and by the time we left she was more content and felt more assured about our future. Also, being now relatively close to England, she could look forward to the possibility of visiting us.

However, after returning to London I began to be plagued by doubts as to whether I should be embarking on a career in medicine. The prospect of five more years before qualification and the likelihood of a further long period of specialisation were daunting, and I had enjoyed my experience with mining exploration in Canada. Also around this time I became much influenced by the philosophy of Albert Camus, and his concept of Man's absurd relationship with the world did not make a decision of this importance any easier. (During the next two years having read all of his books, most of them at least twice, I came to have a much more constructive view of his philosophy and he has remained an important influence throughout my life.) Nevertheless, during this time of indecision I did sufficient work to ensure I would pass the Biology examination, and continued to enjoy my rugby.

Elizabeth had by now given up her psychiatric social work and was teaching at a primary school in London. We saw a lot of each other and enjoyed going to plays and concerts together. I also knew she appreciated being able to talk to me about Dave, and share some of her concerns as to whether she was right to be marrying him. Towards the end of the academic year I began to consider what I might do during the long vacation and it was not long before another summer job in Canada began to seem attractive. When I wrote to my mother about this, explaining that I wanted to experience again what I had enjoyed so much, and to look at a career in medicine from a Canadian perspective, she replied with a passionate letter trying to dissuade me from this, and concluding:

"You are the only English. You may not realise it, but you carry the family's hopes for a life lived to a great tradition. Blessings, great opportunities have been showered on you. Great responsibilities are inevitably also yours. You have a rich inheritance in the men of our family who have gone before you

– your grandfathers, your father, Uncle Max. They would give inspiration to any young man. And in you lie the same gifts, talents, graces. Be true to the hallowed past. Set your gaze high to the future. Rise to your full stature to meet this challenge."

This was the first time my mother had ever put such pressure on me not to follow a course of action I had chosen. And I could only surmise that she thought, correctly, that this would make a decision to remain in medicine more difficult than it already was. Also, having told her about Vieno and that we continued to remain in touch, I suspect she was worried that if I returned to Canada I might end up marrying her. However, after further correspondence I think I was able to dispel some though not all of her concerns. So I wrote to my various contacts in Canada and through one of them managed to secure summer employment with Kennco Exploration (Canada) Ltd. At that time Kennecott was the biggest copper producer in the world and had a tough Australian, Frank Sullivan, as head of their geological activities in Canada. My immediate boss was another Australian, Frank Joklik, and we were to become involved in exploration for copper in Northern Quebec.

I sailed for Canada on the 'Empress of Britain' at the beginning of July and for the next three months I was in charge of small field parties working over a large area north of Rouyn engaged in ground magnetic and electromagnetic surveys, as well as staking new claims for the Company. During the summer we spent time in five different camps and I loved being in the bush again, working in relative isolation so far from civilisation. The main problem was the mosquitoes, which were worse than anything I had experienced in Africa, but fortunately they did not transmit malaria. The weather was also bad much of the time and there were many days when I remained soaked to the skin. Frank Joklik joined me in several of the expeditions and although very different from Frank Mills we soon became firm friends. My thoughts continued to revolve around whether I should continue with medicine or remain in mining but by the end of the summer I felt I should stick with my original decision to become a doctor.

While I was in Canada my mother's time in Ibiza came to an end. She had enjoyed living there and was sad to leave, writing to me that she had left "in a nice flurry of farewells and a real pang of sadness at leaving the kindly, likeable, loveable Spaniards". She went first to Andorra for a short spell and then in August to Jersey where she joined friends from South

Africa and had Elizabeth and Dave to stay for two weeks at the end of the month. During this time she got to know Dave and to appreciate many of his sterling qualities. She could see how happy the two of them were together and consequently felt content about their impending marriage.. It was agreed that Mum would join Elizabeth in London in September and that they would share a flat until the wedding, which had been set for May the next year (1957), after which she would return to South Africa.

I once again returned to England via New York, this time on board the S.S. United States. On my way to New York I stopped at Concord, Massachusetts to visit Gale Robb, whom I had met on the boat going to Canada earlier in the year. During my short stay with her family I was thrilled to be able to meet Ralph Waldo Emerson's grandson, who was a near neighbour, and to tell him what an influence his grandfather had been on me during the preceding two years.

When I arrived back in England I had just turned twenty-four and the next year proved to be the most turbulent and difficult of my life. I had decided not to return to London House and rented a room in Earls Court close to where Elizabeth and my mother were staying. I went to Guy's for lectures and tried to apply myself to the study of Anatomy and Physiology. As the days passed I grew more and more dissatisfied with my lot and depressed at the thought of what lay ahead. And in this state of turmoil I went to see the Dean and told him that I wanted to give up medicine. He observed that I was old enough to know my own mind and that was that. It all had a rather dreamlike quality about it as I had no clear thought as to what path my future should take. I would have liked to leave London immediately but agreed to my mother's request that I should remain with them until after Elizabeth's wedding. I took to spending much time in my room reading voraciously and also became engaged in a brief but passionate affair with an attractive and artistic woman six years older than me, who rejoiced in the delightful name of Pandora. She helped me think through a few of my more difficult problems and also dissuaded me from embarking on some of my wilder schemes, such as joining the Hungarian Freedom Fighters – this being the time of the Hungarian revolution. Understandably both my mother and Elizabeth were concerned by my lack of direction and I was encouraged to find at least temporary employment, which I finally did with the '1820s Settlers' Association'. They had offices near Trafalgar Square opposite South Africa House and were engaged with interviewing and providing information to potential emigrants to South Africa and the newly formed Federation of Rhodesia and Nyasaland. I recall a difficult visit to Glasgow, where I had great difficulty understanding the broad Glaswegian accent, followed by the same problem the next day when I was in Belfast. I had kept in touch with Frank Joklik who was aware of my circumstances, and in January he offered me employment with Kennco from May for an exploration project they were planning in the Ungava peninsula, this being in the northern-most part of Quebec Province just south of Baffin Island. This fitted in with the timing of Elizabeth's wedding and I was pleased to accept it as offering some security while I made up my mind what to do with my life, one possibility being to take an MSc in Geology at the end of the summer.

During the ensuing months I began to have grave doubts that my decision to give up medicine had been wrong. I returned to the view that I wanted a job that had meaning both for me and for others, and also the satisfaction of being able to look back across a life and see some tangible accomplishments for the common good. But the problem remained of how to achieve this. One redeeming feature of this period was that I felt I was providing help and support to Elizabeth, who was having occasional doubts herself about her impending marriage. I should add that these were quite unwarranted as she and Dave have now enjoyed more than fifty years of a very happy marriage. Their wedding took place on 13th April 1957 and was a short and simple affair in the Kensington Registry Office. It was attended by Dave's mother and brother, Peter, and by my mother and me. We then had a good lunch at a local restaurant, after which Elizabeth and Dave departed for their honeymoon in Cornwall and the Augers returned to Southampton. I remained for a short time in London, during which I saw as much of my mother as possible, and then by the beginning of May I was back in Canada, sharing an apartment with Frank Joklik in Quebec City, while we prepared for the expedition to Ungava.

I think the new environment and the ability to discuss thoughts and ideas freely with Frank helped to crystallise the view that I had made a serious mistake in giving up medicine. Initially, when considering this, I assumed there was no chance of ever being readmitted to Guy's but now I decided that I could not proceed without exploring this possibility. So in early June I wrote the following letter to the Dean:

"Dear Sir,

Last October, shortly after starting my second year at Guy's, I decided to give up my medical studies and at an interview with you on 17th October I informed you of my decision. I told myself then that I no longer wanted to be a doctor and that it would be wiser for me to continue with the profession that I was already qualified in.

Looking back on it I can see that apart from being in an unsettled state of mind my action was predominantly a result of impatience and weakness. On the one hand I could see years of hard study ahead; on the other a job which already offered substantial financial rewards.

Soon after leaving I began to apprehend the full meaning of my loss and on occasions I came close to asking for re-admittance to the School. But then I also felt that I had made my decision and that I could not expect other than to remain with it. However, as the days go by I realise ever more strongly that it is medicine that I want to do. This decision, born during my third year at University in South Africa, has I think always been with me. But previously I would not recognise the fact that anything worthwhile in life could not, of necessity, be achieved with ease.

So I write now and ask you to consider my case compassionately. I realise that my conduct so far has not been such as to warrant a sympathetic reaction, but I do ask you to give serious consideration to my plea. On my part, all I can offer is the assurance that, if given the opportunity of recommencing my studies at Guy's, I would do everything in my power to be worthy of the trust shown.

I know that it will require discipline and industry and that it will involve certain sacrifices. But I feel sincerely that my desire to be a doctor is now mature and strong enough to enable me to achieve the goal. I ask you to have faith in this.

Yours faithfully, Terence English"

A fortnight later I received a reply from the Dean, Dr George Houston. It was brief and to the point, concluding: "given the circumstances, we are prepared to re-admit you to your studies." I have often pondered about the enormous impact that decision has had on my life. Had it gone the other way, I would never have enjoyed the great satisfaction that I eventually derived from my years as a surgeon in the National Health Service. And it gave me great pleasure, when I met George Houston many years later at a Guy's function, when I was President of the Royal College of Surgeons of England, to thank him once again for so generously placing his trust in me. Two years later, by a strange quirk of fate we met again – this time in Southwark Cathedral – when he and I were both awarded Honorary Fellowships of the United Medical and Dental Schools of Guy's and St Thomas's Hospitals.

With this behind me, and feeling at last fully committed to medicine, my mood lifted and I was able to enjoy the next three months in Canada with pleasure and a sense of optimism about the future. My mother was overjoyed when she heard the news and Elizabeth wrote:

"The immediate impact of it hit me silently and slowly in the solar plexus. But it is wonderful news. It is not an easy road you have chosen. Frustration, disillusionment, maybe even moments of despair, but I hope with all my heart that you will find rewards you have not even dreamed of, and a fulfilment."

By the end of June plans for the Ungava project were complete and Frank and I headed north, first to Fort Chimo, a small Eskimo (Inuit) settlement on the banks of the Koksoak river and then on to the concession we were to survey for Kennco. We lived in small tents and had the help of two experienced prospectors, one of whom acted as cook.

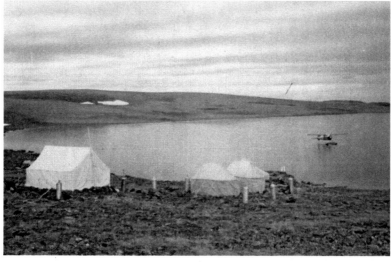

Our camp in Ungava. Summer 1957

We were now well beyond the tree line and the country was undulating and barren but with sufficient outcrop of rocks to facilitate our geological mapping. At times the wind was fierce but we didn't mind this because while it lasted it suppressed the ubiquitous mosquitoes. We had a strenuous life and I reckoned that we covered over 600 miles on foot during the short time we were there. By mid-August the days were already turning cold and we had the first fine snow of approaching winter. The geese were in migration and great winging formations of them were to be seen against the stormy skies. The Loons alone remained faithful, and I loved their eerie, haunting cries that would come across the lake near our camp. For me these birds will always symbolise the purity and vastness of the Ungava plains and I used to thrill to their cry in the early mornings and again in the evenings as the light faded shimmering over the water of the nearby lake.

By early September our field work was done but before returning to Fort Chimo Frank and I flew to the Eskimo village of Sugluk on the shores of the Hudson Strait to tell them where our camp was and that we were leaving some provisions and equipment there which we would like them to have.

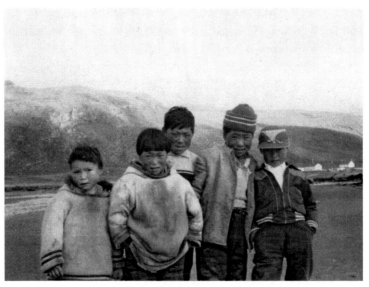

Eskimo children at Sugluk.

They were delighted with this and in return gave each of us a fine example of their sculpture. Mine is of an Eskimo hunter with a large bear slung over his shoulder and this still provides me with a precious memory of our time in Ungava. Another event to be remembered occurred on our last night at Fort Chimo when I went outside before turning in and found the Northern Lights blazing away like a dancing green curtain, tinted with bright pink streaks across the north western sky. The splendour and vastness of my wild surroundings merged with a deep gratitude that I had been re-accepted by Guy's and a determination to give of my best when I returned.

After getting back to Quebec City Frank and I completed the process of mapping the results of our field work and writing a report on the project. I then returned to England on the 'Empress of England', arriving back in London on 30th September where I was met by a delighted and relieved mother. I chose to return to London House because I thought it would be more conducive to hard study and re-started my 2nd MB on my 25th birthday. I now immersed myself in the study of Anatomy and Physiology and recognising these pre-clinical studies as being the big hurdle decided

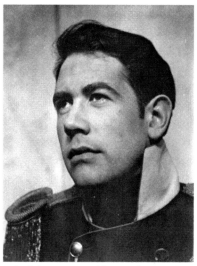

As Montserrat. November 1957.

to give up rugby until I had passed the examinations, which were due in eighteen months. At that time, anatomy was still taught in great detail, with dissection of the human body being an important part of the course. I recall the first time I was faced with dissecting a cadaver, thinking of it as having once been human with the hopes, frustrations and desires that are our lot. But this soon passed as we steadily dissected and displayed the various parts on which we would be regularly tested. I worked hard and it was with great satisfaction that I saw my name at the top of the 'Vivas' list at the end of the first term, and this despite having been encouraged to take a leading part in the play "Montserrat", which took place towards the end of that term.

The latter indicates that I didn't become entirely devoted to my studies and to add to the pleasure of life I bought a 1930 Rolls Royce for the magnificent sum of £175. I reasoned this was justified on the basis of what I had earned in Canada during the previous three summers. Having missed a year, I was now with a different group of students and by the beginning of the new year (1958) I had become fond of a stunningly beautiful Indian girl in our class. Sheela's father ran a general practice near Guy's and she and her brother and sister had all been born and educated in London. Our relationship took time to develop but during the next three years we became deeply attached to each other.

My mother returned to South Africa at the end of 1957 but Elizabeth still had another year in London before she and Dave emigrated to Rhodesia. He was away at sea a lot and as usual we found strength and comfort in each other's company. I decided to spend yet one more summer in Canada during the next long vacation and was pleased to be able to arrange employment once again with Kennco. So I continued to work hard until the end of June, when I flew to New York via 'Icelandic Airways' and then travelled by bus to Montreal before joining Frank Joklik for more geophysical work. This took place in Northern Quebec but in an area not as remote as Ungava. For much of the time I was on my own apart from two prospectors with whom I had worked previously. Jack Lusko was a large rather morose Polish man and Robert Guay a volatile French Canadian. They did not get on well together and we had no cook so it was not an altogether happy camp. But I was kept busy with an electromagnetic survey and some geochemical assaying of stream sediments, using the small laboratory kit I had taken with me. I also had to join Jack and Robert with quite a lot of the axe work, cutting lines through the woods for the survey grid. During the short season we were flown into no fewer than four different camps while Frank was supervising the drilling on nearby claims. I enjoyed the work, but this time had the peace of mind of knowing where my future lay, as evidenced by a letter to my mother in which I wrote:

"I think a lot about medicine and, oh Mum, I'm glad, glad that I took the decision last year to return to it. I have the conviction now that it is going to offer me untold interest and that I will also be suited to the work. And I don't really regret not having started it sooner, for I have learned a lot during these 8½ years since leaving school."

After return to London I continued to work hard for the last six months prior to the 2nd MB examinations. Despite this I remained concerned about the possibility of failing and must have transmitted this to my mother, who wrote to me shortly before the examinations:

"But I – and everyone who loves you – and there are many my dearest – will hold strongly to the conviction that you will <u>not</u> know failure, and that your lucky star will be shining strong and serene – even if it's behind the fog and clouds of a London sky. Keep a clear head and a stout heart and you will not fail."

As it was, of the 76 who sat the exam, 43 passed all the papers and I was one of these. The relief was immense and now I could begin the clinical training that I had looked forward to ever since I had started at Guy's

At this stage the class was divided in two and I was attached as ward-clerk to a surgical firm for three months. Before departing for Canada the previous year I had sold my Rolls in order to pay for the airfare but I now bought another. This time it was a 1923 Rolls Royce Landaulette by Barker, for which I paid £40. It was rather battered, having done many hundreds of thousands of miles but was still mechanically sound and was much admired by my fellow medical students. The Porters at Guy's also found it amusing and would sometimes let me park it in the forecourt amongst the smarter and much younger Rolls driven by some of the consultants. By this time I had become good friends with a younger student in our class, James Carmichael, and he and I decided to try and get a labouring job during the short summer holiday. We set our sights on Trawsfynydd in North Wales where we heard work had just started on a nuclear power station. So we set off in the Rolls, and after a leisurely journey arrived at the site the next day. There we were met by the foreman of a gang of a dozen Welsh labourers who were engaged in digging a large trench as part of the foundations. He took one look at us, another at the car, and declared that there were no jobs going. We protested that we had come all the way from London, having been informed by his Head Office that labourers were indeed needed and after further persuasion he agreed to take us on for the next four weeks. So we secured lodgings in nearby Ffestiniogg and used to drive out to the site each day when we would park the Rolls near the trench, collect our picks and shovels and start digging. Our fellow labourers, some of whom had little English, initially regarded us as being very odd but with time barriers were broken down and we came to enjoy each others company. That summer of 1959 was amongst the best on record, with days of unbroken sunshine except when we climbed Snowdon on a dark and misty day. We enjoyed the physical demands of digging the trench and soon became very fit. This was as well, because having got the hurdle of 2nd MB behind me I had decided to resume playing rugby, at least for the next two years.

The clinical period at Guy's was divided into attachments of three months, during which we rotated through the various specialties, with two each at different levels of seniority in medicine and surgery. During these we became part of a 'Firm' consisting usually of two consultants, a senior registrar, registrar and houseman (Pre-registration House Officer). Guy's prided itself on the extent of clinical experience it provided for its students and much of our time was spent on the wards clerking patients. This involved taking their medical history and examining them prior to the case being discussed on a ward round, which were conducted by both consultants and registrars. Most consultant ward rounds were formal affairs. The Great Man – and they were nearly all men – would usually be met on the front steps of the hospital by his senior registrar, registrar and houseman, and then be conducted to one of his wards. There he would join the sister of that ward and the medical students. The entourage would then proceed around each patient with the students presenting the history, physical signs and investigations of each new patient before the differential diagnosis was discussed. The consultant might then go on to teach on the disease and treatment relevant to that patient. I regarded this, and still do, as an excellent way of teaching medical students. We were exposed to a wide variety of medical and surgical conditions, which could be related to specific patients rather than just learning about these in a book. We also acquired, through the example of our seniors, valuable attitudes and professional behaviour in dealing with patients. The firm structure also contributed to continuity of care, which is of such importance for the welfare of patients and which has now been so sadly eroded by the European Working Time Directive.

Besides the ward work we were expected to read up the literature relevant to the firm we were on and on which we would subsequently be tested. In addition there were regular lunchtime lectures by the teaching staff and these were mostly of a high standard. Unlike today, there were also regular post-mortem demonstrations, which again were held during lunchtime. These were usually conducted by the famous forensic pathologist, Keith Simpson. He was a great showman and taught us much morbid pathology, always linking his findings to the clinical features of the relevant disease. So that if, for example, the patient had died of a heart attack, he would talk about the likely symptoms associated with this and then demonstrate the narrowings in the coronary arteries and how these were responsible for the damage to the heart muscle.

I enjoyed each rotation as they came. One of the more unusual ones was Obstetrics and Gynaecology, during which we spent a fortnight delivering babies on 'The District', this being the surrounding area of Bermondsey and Southwark. This service was for mothers who had been followed up in the antenatal clinic and judged safe to have a home birth. As students we were always accompanied by a midwife. It was important to reach an agreement with her beforehand, as on entering the house the family would often assume that you were the doctor, whereas in truth one was very dependent on the midwife to see you through the delivery. A tricky situation, which if handled properly, resulted in joy and satisfaction all round.

Towards the end of 1959 I decided the time had come to leave London House and started looking for a place of my own. I was lucky to find a delightful sub-basement flat in St Leonard's Terrace in Chelsea, which I rented from the Foord-Kelseys who occupied the house above. This comprised a bed-sitting room, small kitchen and bathroom, all for the modest rent of £8 per week and could not have suited me better. Not far from the river it was also close to the King's Road and Sloane Square. Then, on the 16th December I heard the shocking news of my mother's sudden death in a car accident. She had been staying with her sister Doreen, in Underberg, Natal, and the two of them were driving to Pietermaritzburg when the car went out of control as they were descending a steep pass. My mother, who was driving, was thrown out and killed immediately, whereas Doreen rolled down the hillside within the car and escaped with minor injuries. I flew out as soon as I could, arriving in time for a solemn Christmas in Underberg where many of the family had gathered, including Dave and Elizabeth. It was a dreadful shock to us all as my mother was only 63 and in excellent health and full of vitality. I tried to draw some comfort from her oft repeated declaration that she didn't want to live beyond being of help to her family and many friends. And also, that she had lived to see her beloved daughter happily married with her first child having been born three months earlier, and with me finally on my way to becoming a doctor. She was a most remarkable person in her capacity for love and friendship and in turn was loved by so many people from a wide spectrum of background.

Returning to London I remained intermittently depressed for several months, despite the busy days at Guy's and the demands of rugby. What added to this was that while I was in South Africa, Sheela had finally told her parents about our relationship and their reaction was such that I think she realised that we could never marry. I also knew that in South Africa so called "mixed marriages" were illegal under the prevailing apartheid laws – and remained so for the next 30 years – so that this would bar me from returning there. To take my mind off these sombre thoughts, I once again became deeply committed to rugby and it was with huge pride, and not a little apprehension, that I was elected Captain of the 1st XV at the end of the season. However, I was fortunate in being able to take a strong team into the next year. The forwards were particularly powerful and included Stan Cooke, who was now an anatomy demonstrator, Barry Blackwell, the previous year's Captain, Bill Treadwell, a future English international, and John Hockey, a Cambridge 'Blue'. Guy's prided itself on being one of the oldest Rugby Clubs in the world and at the time we regularly turned out five XVs every Saturday. The 1st XV had a good season, at the end of which we had the great satisfaction of winning the Inter-Hospitals Cup by beating St Thomas's, the favourites in the Final With this behind me, and only one year to go before final examinations, I decided that my rugby-playing days should come to an end.

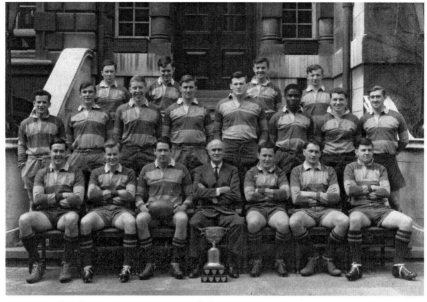

Guy's 1st XV. Winners of the Inter-Hospitals Cup. 1961.

That final year as a student passed happily and smoothly. I enjoyed living in Chelsea and the clinical work became increasingly interesting. During the last medical firm I particularly enjoyed the cardiology component and decided that this would be my preferred option when applying for pre-registration house jobs. A number of us had decided to sit both the Conjoint Examination (MRCS; LRCP) given by the Royal Colleges of Surgeons and Physicians, and the London University MB examination. The former was taken in stages and if successful allowed one to qualify three months earlier and hence start 'house jobs' that much sooner. This appealed to me and, having successfully passed 'Conjoint' in January 1962, I decided that a short holiday in South Africa was indicated before starting internship, I hoped at Guy's, in March. So I went first to Swaziland to see Elizabeth and Dave at Ubombo ranches, where he was chief engineer and Elizabeth had just had her second child earlier that month, and then on to Natal to spend a short time with my Uncle Max and Aunt Doreen. I loved being back in what I still regarded as my homeland, and amongst family that had always meant so much to me. Soon after I returned to London the list of 'house jobs' starting on 1st March was published and I was delighted to see that I had got my first choice. This was for three months as Assistant House Surgeon (AHS) to Mr Rex Lawrie. I had planned it this way, as after the next three months as a Casualty Officer I hoped to spend the last six as House Physician to the senior Cardiologist, Dr Charles Baker. So by the beginning of March I had moved out of my flat, sold the Rolls and taken up residence in the 'College' at Guy's, which was reserved for resident house staff and which became my home for the next eighteen months. My salary was £600 pa plus board and lodging and my transition from mining to medicine was now complete. The new career was about to begin.

Chapter 4
Surgical Training and Marriage

Pre-registration House Officer

There were four surgical firms at Guy's, each staffed by a senior and a junior consultant surgeon. The latter though nominally 'junior' were already very experienced and throughout one week in every four their half of the firm was responsible for all surgical emergencies admitted to the hospital. However, they knew that when their colleague retired they would become senior surgeon and be absolved of further emergency work. A senior registrar and registrar served both surgeons and each consultant had either a House Surgeon (HS) or an Assistant House Surgeon (AHS). Our firm comprised Sir Hedley Atkins, Professor of Surgery, and Rex Lawrie. My duties were strictly with Mr Lawrie for whom I soon developed an immense respect. Although very clever, he was innately modest, almost self-deprecating, and perhaps because of this never received the wider professional recognition he deserved. He was a very fast surgeon and a superb teacher and mentor and his many trainees soon came to appreciate his vast knowledge of both medicine and surgery. Unlike many consultants of his era he would patiently and often humorously assist his trainees through operations, something I benefited greatly from when four years later I became his RSO (Resident Surgical Officer) at the Bolingbroke Hospital in Wandsworth. He frequently challenged conventional surgical practice and made learning both a serious business and fun.

After an interesting and stimulating three months I moved on to become a Casualty Officer. This was an entirely different experience. We worked in shifts with no on-call duties and were therefore able to enjoy some welcome time off. When on duty we saw a wide range of medical and surgical conditions, some trivial, some life threatening. Being still inexperienced we needed at times to be able to call on more senior colleagues. During the day the consultant in charge of the department was often present. Otherwise one had to contact the on-call House Physician or House Surgeon, who would then decide whether admission was indicated or not. Occasionally if confronted by what appeared to be a serious emergency one would get the whole on-call team down immediately. This all provided excellent general experience, and sensibly at this time the requirements for sitting the final FRCS examination included six months in a Casualty Department.

I then began my last pre-registration appointment as House Physician (HP) to Drs Charles Baker and Charles Joiner. Dr Baker was both general physician and senior cardiologist and it was because of my developing interest in this specialty that I applied for the job. Dr Joiner had just published a successful textbook of medicine and to students appeared to be a walking encyclopaedia on all matters medical. He seemed, however, to have been somewhat soured by the inordinately long time he had served as a senior registrar before becoming a consultant at Guy's, and could treat his juniors harshly if errors of diagnosis or treatment were made.

Despite this, I enjoyed my six months on the firm immensely. I loved seeing new admissions with the medical students and developed a genuine sense of 'ownership' of the male and female patients in our two wards, which I would always visit last thing at night. I was also fortunate in having two very good registrars to support me. Tony Trafford was the senior, later to become Minister of State for Health in the Lords in Margaret Thatcher's government, and Anthony Hopkins was the registrar who became a distinguished neurologist. I also got on well with the Senior Registrar in the Cardiac department, Hywel Davies, who became a life-long friend and later gave up his practice in Denver, Colorado, to join me at Papworth as cardiologist to the transplant programme when one was very much needed.

I developed the utmost regard for Charles Baker, who was both a caring and a fine physician. At the time he was an elderly bachelor but a few years later surprised everyone when he married Jean Bailey, who was the delightful lady who looked after the 'College' in which all of us residents lived. Towards the end of my time on the firm I discussed my future with both of my chiefs. Dr Baker was pleased when he heard that I wished to pursue a career in cardiology and suggested that a good next step would be to spend six months with the cardiac surgeons "to see what they were up to". This appealed to me but I wasn't sure whether Sir Russell Brock, as

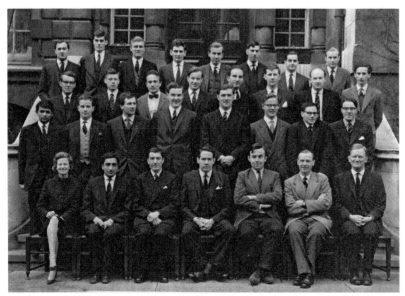
Guy's Hospital Residents, 1963.

he then was, would look favourably on having a would-be cardiologist to train rather than a surgeon. However, Dr Baker said he would look into the matter. When I approached Charles Joiner the response was different. He asked how old I was and when I replied that I was thirty he declared I was too old to think of specialising and should rather go into General Practice. I regarded this as unnecessarily discouraging and having pursued Dr Baker's suggestion was delighted when I was appointed Senior House Officer (SHO) to the Thoracic Unit at Guy's with a start date three months later on 1st June 1963. When I bumped into Charles Joiner at a Guy's Biennial Dinner in 1973 I couldn't resist telling him that ten years earlier he had given me some bad advice and that I would like him to know that I had just been appointed consultant cardiothoracic surgeon to Papworth and Addenbrooke's Hospitals. His response was to walk away without uttering a word.

Holiday in South Africa
By the end of a long winter, during which I hardly left the hospital, I was ready for a holiday. That winter was also to be remembered for the last bad 'smog' to be suffered by London, during which we were kept immensely busy with large numbers of patients with chronic bronchitis being admitted in respiratory failure. I therefore decided to use some of the intervening time before starting on the Thoracic Unit to visit South Africa.

I decided to fly there and back via the cheapest means and this turned out to be with Trek Airways. They owned two elderly DC4s that used to travel in tandem between Luxembourg and Johannesburg. The planes flew at about 10,000 feet so as passengers you had a good view of Africa as it unfolded beneath you. Each aircraft was serviced by a single crew, so that the journey had to be divided into four short sections with three overnight stops. I found this leisurely progression a good way to travel, providing as it did lots of interest along the way. One such event happened on my return journey. We were flying over the Sahara desert when the air hostess, as they were then called, asked for a doctor to attend to a passenger who was in difficulty at the front of the aircraft. Having proudly entered my name as "Dr English" on the passenger list I felt I had to offer my services and was led to a rather fat German lady who was having a panic attack. She was over-breathing to the extent that she had developed tetany, which resulted in her fingers curling up in spasm and only served to increase her distress. Having made the diagnosis I embarked on the traditional treatment. This involved calling for a large brown paper bag, into which I encouraged her to re-breathe. This had to be done through an interpreter and was observed with interest by the passengers nearby, during which I could sense an increasing degree of skepticism. However, with persistence the level of expired carbon dioxide in the bag, which was then rebreathed, was sufficient to increase the level of ionised calcium in the blood and thereby relieve the tetany. Having achieved this rather unexpected result the lady calmed down and as I returned to my seat at the back of the aircraft I was greeted with a prolonged burst of applause, similar to that which might have been awarded to a magician who had just pulled a rabbit out of a hat. Furthermore that night, as a token of Trek's appreciation, the Captain booked me into the Nile Hilton in Cairo, which until then was quite the smartest hotel I had ever stayed in.

There were no such problems on the way out and after landing in Johannesburg I went first to the Midlands of Natal to visit my Lund cousins and to stay with Aunt Doreen in Underberg. Then to Max in Pietermaritzburg who was interested to hear about my experience as a house officer at Guy's and that I was about to embark on six months of surgery, albeit as a means towards a career in cardiology. However, the main attraction for the visit was an invitation from my sister Elizabeth to join her and Dave and their good friends Marge and Gordon Grange for a holiday at Plettenberg Bay, where they had rented a house near the sea for the first two weeks of April. This proved to be an idyllic holiday. Plettenberg Bay– or Plet as the locals know it – was then a charming small village with some beautiful beaches to swim from and great walks nearby. These included one around the Robberg Peninsula, which jutted out into the Indian Ocean along the southern side of the Bay, and which soon became my favourite.

Engagement to Ann

Uncle Fred, my father's middle brother, who normally lived in a remote area near Cape St Francis, happened to be looking after a house in nearby Knysna and having made contact with him he was keen to introduce Elizabeth and me to his friends Gwen and Mordaunt Dicey, who were farming at Wittedrif, not far from Plettenberg Bay. So a visit was arranged and there we met Mordaunt, his son Tom and his daughter Ann. Gwen was in the Orange Free State staying with her other daughter, Mary, who had just given birth to a son. Mordaunt was the eldest of seven sons and his father, Leicester Dicey, had started the Cape Orchard Company at Hex River Valley in the 1890s, at which time refrigeration had made it possible to send export grapes to the markets in London. All seven sons had joined their father farming in the Hex River Valley but Mordaunt later left to restore the fortunes of the Smartt Syndicate farms in the Northern Cape, which had been started by his father-in-law, Sir Thomas Smartt. When he retired he bought the farm 'Lawn' at Wittendrif from where he would indulge in his passion for fishing from Robberg. Tom had joined him to establish the pastures for sheep and the dams for irrigation and then took over running the farm for his parents. Ann, who had trained as a nurse at Groote Schuur hospital in Cape Town, was at home to run the house while her mother was in the Free State.

Fred had been life-long friends with the family and my mother had stayed at 'Lawn' on her way through the Garden Route some years before her death and written to me about how much she had enjoyed the visit, so that when Elizabeth, Dave and I were taken to meet the family there were already many connections. I was immediately attracted to Ann and after a very happy afternoon I arranged to meet her the next day in Plet. We soon fell in love and when Liz and Dave returned to Swaziland a few days later I decided to remain in Plet so that I could see more of her and was delighted when I was invited to stay at 'Lawn'. During the next week Ann and I were with each other more or less constantly, either on the farm, meeting her friends or exploring the surrounding countryside. I immediately warmed to Tom and came to respect and admire Mordaunt despite his rather stern demeanour. By the end of the week I could delay my visit to Cape Town no longer and on the last evening before supper I proposed to Ann as we were walking back to the house along the tree-lined avenue. She was overcome and pleaded a few hours in which to make up her mind but her decision was cast within half an hour. I was then able to approach her father who was clearly pleased with the prospect and readily gave us his blessing.

The plan was that I would complete my six months on the Thoracic Unit and then return to Plettenberg Bay at the end of November when we would marry. In the meantime I was due to spend a week in the Cardiac Unit at Groote Schuur where Donald Ross had suggested I visit his friend Christiaan Barnard to see what he was up to, the two of them having qualified at the same time from Cape Town University. En route I stopped off at Knysna to tell Fred that I had become engaged to Ann and he was overjoyed with the news. Then on to spend a night at Robertson with my godmother Aunt Violet who, as a particularly close friend of Gwen's, was equally delighted and who soon spread the news far and wide amongst the family.

I had an interesting week at Groote Schuur during which I was able to attend the theatre and watch Barnard operate. At that time he was relatively unknown although his results in congenital heart disease could compare with the best in the world. He was obsessional about every aspect of an operation and the patient's aftercare, even to the extent of requiring his experienced registrar to spend the whole of the first night with the patient in the intensive care cubicle monitoring the blood pressure and vital signs. He was very short tempered and would shout at his assistants if things were not going well, so that the atmosphere in theatre was always tense. I also spent time with Robert Frater, another Cape Town graduate, who had done his cardiac surgical training at the Mayo Clinic in Rochester, Minnesota, and then returned to a consultant post at Groote Schuur shortly after Barnard had taken over as chief. Bob seemed to me a more mature and technically better surgeon and during the next year it became apparent that Cape Town was not big enough for both of them so he accepted a job at the Albert Einstein hospital in New York where he had a distinguished career.

While in Cape Town I kept in touch with Ann by telephone and it was agreed that I should visit her mother before leaving South Africa. Gwen

Dicey, as mentioned, was staying with Mary who had married Charles Johnstone who was running a large farm in the Orange Free State. I would then make a quick trip to Swaziland to share my thoughts with Elizabeth, after which Ann would come to Johannesburg to say goodbye before I returned to England. Violet had generously offered me her car to do the journey in. However, when I went to Robertson to collect it she decided she could not miss the opportunity of coming with me as far as the Free State where she would stay with Gwen, Mary and Charles until I returned from my trip to Swaziland. She was always a good storyteller and made a wonderful companion on the long journey north. In retrospect I wished I had been able to record some of her wilder accounts, which included tiger-hunting in India when she and Gwen's sister, Dodie, had gone to visit my Uncle Henry who had moved there after the First World War and was coffee-planting in South India. There were also interesting tales about early days in Robertson where she grew up, and about her experience as a teacher in pre-war Rhodesia.

Gwen was kind and gracious and made me feel welcome as a new addition to the family. She also gave me two magnificent diamonds set in a brooch, which she generously suggested might be incorporated in an engagement ring for Ann. These had been personally chosen by Cecil Rhodes as a gift to her mother, Lady Smartt, Sir Thomas having first been Rhodes' personal physician and then later his political colleague. One of my early school friends, David Greig, had taken over his father's well-known jewellery business in Johannesburg, so en route to Swaziland I called to see him. After admiring the quality of the diamonds, he said that he would find an equally fine sapphire to set between them. He was as good as his word and I was able to give Ann her beautiful engagement ring when she came to Johannesburg for a brief visit prior to my departure. We spent two very happy days together whilst staying with my other godmother, Mary Bell, and then it was time for me to board Trek Airways for the flight back to England.

Senior House Officer on Guy's Thoracic Unit
Soon after my return I was once again ensconced in the College at Guy's and began a job that caused me to follow a new Star, leading to the most important decision of my medical career. Cardiac surgery in 1963 was at a fascinating stage of its development. Gross in Boston (1938) and Crafoord in Sweden (1944) had led the way on operations on major vessels close to the heart. They were followed by Bailey and Harken in the USA

and Brock in Britain who performed 'closed' operations on the heart itself for the relief of mitral stenosis. This involved introducing dilators into the heart to open up the narrowed mitral valve. However, by the early 1950s it had become clear that further advances could only be achieved if a means could be found to stop the heart safely for long enough to enable defects within its interior to be repaired under direct vision. This led to the development of the heart-lung machine, or pump-oxygenator as it came to be called. This was first used successfully by John Gibbon in Philadelphia on 6th May 1953. However, his next two patients died so he left it to others to take forward this exciting new technology. Foremost amongst these was John Kirklin at the Mayo Clinic, who refined the Gibbons machine and then, in March 1955 began the world's first open heart programme using a heart-lung machine. Interestingly, during the preceding year and only 50 miles away in Minneapolis, Walton Lillehei was embarking on an incredible series of open heart operations on children, in which the mother or father was used as a human pump-oxygenator by temporarily connecting their respective venous and arterial systems to the child to support the circulation while the heart was

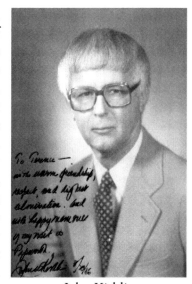

John Kirklin

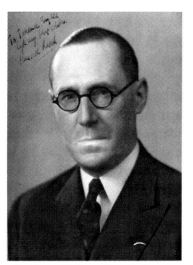

Sir Russell (later Lord) Brock, 1963.

stopped. The rationale for this was that morbidity from the early heart-lung machines was high, but as Lillehei's critics pointed out, the potential for an operation to result in the death of both child and parent was unlikely to last and indeed steady improvements in the components of pump-oxygenators meant that many cardiac surgical units were soon embarked upon open-heart operations. This was true of Guy's where Brock had been early in the field and when I joined the Thoracic Unit he was at the height of his powers and about to become President of the Royal College of Surgeons. Difficult, and at times impossibly demanding, those who worked for him seldom resented his barrage of criticism. Perhaps this was because he imposed such high standards on his own performance, which he frequently failed to achieve technically, and which no doubt was the source of much of his frustration. But at the same time no one could fail to recognise the power of his vision or the genius of his clinical skills. He also knew only too well the disappointments and failures endured whilst pioneering this new specialty, as evidenced by this extract from an article he wrote in 1962:

"The only answer to those grim moments when great despair and at times real and severe anguish are felt is to have faith in our basic policy and decisions. I do not mean that we should not seek out errors and adjust them, but tenacity of purpose is essential."

Donald Ross, who had previously been Sir Russell's senior registrar and who had only recently been appointed to the consultant staff, provided a complimentary range of talents. He never got rattled, his technical skills were unsurpassed, and his capacity for innovation brought the whole range of cardiac surgery within his ambit. It was a hugely interesting and exciting team to be part of, and I soon began to question whether I should not devote my future to cardiac surgery rather than cardiology. Having qualified as an engineer, I had an understanding of the mechanical aspects of the heart-lung machine and the design of artificial heart valves that were then

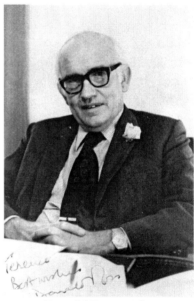

Donald Ross, 1963.

beginning to come into general use. And the heart itself, when displayed at operation, seemed a more interesting organ than any other in the human body. So to be able to enter it and correct congenital defects or replace damaged valves seemed a fascinating path to pursue. The six months passed quickly and towards the end I consulted Brock about my future. In his forthright way he defined how much more demanding was the life of a surgeon as compared with that of a physician, and that cardiac surgery was amongst the most difficult of the surgical specialties. He pointed out that it also offered the opportunity of becoming a really good clinician, as one had the advantage of being able to verify the pathology as seen at operation with the pre-operative diagnosis. In essence he was encouraging but emphasised that it would involve a long and arduous period of training, as I would first have to gain the requisite experience in general surgery and pass the FRCS examination, before embarking on a further five or six years of cardiothoracic training. However, I felt this would be worth it and having also gained the support of Donald Ross I decided that this was what I should do. I then went to see Dr Baker to let him know I would not be returning to cardiology and, as anticipated, he was most understanding. Two immensely important decisions had been made within the year.

Wedding at Plettenberg Bay

Meanwhile Ann and I had kept in communication and preparations for the wedding were hotting up at Plettenberg Bay. The date had been set for 23rd November and my plan was to go first to Pietermaritzberg where, much to my pleasure, Max had offered to drive me to the Cape with Liz, Dave and Jenny, and Corinne and her family, following in their cars. So the convoy set off, stopping en route at Slutterheim to see Henry who was unable to attend the wedding. However, the English side of the family was well represented by Fred, Elsabe, Maud and Violet. We arrived in Plet on the 21st November and booked into the Beacon Island Hotel. Interestingly my mother and father had spent part of their honeymoon there forty years earlier when the previous hotel was still in use. I then went straight to 'Lawn' to be with my excited bride-to-be after which I finalised plans for a party at the hotel for family and special guests on the night before the wedding. This duly went ahead and was in full swing until at about 10 pm the news came through that President Kennedy had been assassinated, which put an abrupt stop to further celebrations.

The next afternoon Ann and I were married by the Bishop of George in the beautiful St Peter's Church overlooking Plettenberg Bay. Mary Johnstone, Ann's sister-in-law, was bridesmaid and my cousin Jack Swan best man, and it was a very happy occasion, marred only by the absence of my parents. The reception was held in the Beacon Island Hotel after which Ann and I drove off in Tom's pick-up truck to the fishing-hut on Robberg, which had been lent to us by the Reids for the first part of our honeymoon. We spent a happy week there, with only one visitor – Hjalmar Thesen from Knysna – and then stayed with Violet in Robertson and John, Ann's younger brother, at Hex River before going on to Natal to visit family there and then back to England in time for Christmas.

Before leaving for South Africa I had found what I believed would be suitable accommodation for us in Blackheath. I thought the Heath and Greenwich Park nearby would appeal to Ann and it was also convenient for Guy's as I had

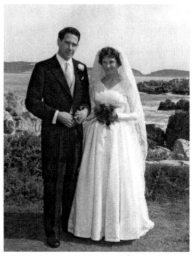

Marriage to Ann – Plettenberg Bay, 23 November 1963.

decided that my next step, if possible, would be to get a job as an anatomy demonstrator in preparation for taking the Primary FRCS examination. Our relatively self-contained flat comprised the ground floor of a house owned by Olive Wright, a retired school teacher, who shared it with her friend Helen Cockburn who taught music at Blackheath's Girls High School and they soon became known as 'Miss Olive' and 'Miss Helen'. They became good friends and during the ensuing years provided good company for Ann during the many nights and days that I was on duty in various hospitals.

Ann and I settled into married life in 40 Vanbrugh Fields, which became our home for the next six years. I managed to get a four months appointment as Casualty Officer at Lewisham Hospital which with my previous experience at Guy's, fulfilled the necessary requirement for the FRCS examination. Following this I got a job as Anatomy demonstrator at Guy's. This did not come easily as when I went to see Professor Warwick, with whom I thought I had got on reasonably well during my 2nd MB studies, he surprised me by saying that under no circumstances would he have me in his department. When I enquired as to the reason he replied that he thought I had been a bad influence on some of the younger students. I felt this was untrue and unjust and sought Sir Russell's help in trying to clarify the situation. I do not know what passed between them but was relieved when, a few weeks later, Professor Warwick informed me that there would be a vacancy for me in two months time on 1st May 1964.

It was fortuitous that I was able to start our marriage doing these two jobs as they allowed Ann and me to enjoy a more settled way of life than later when on-call duties became very disruptive. However, this was not always reflected in a calm and harmonious state of mind on my part. As a result of the haste with which we had become engaged and then married we hardly knew each other and our circumstances now were very different from those we had enjoyed in South Africa. I found that it was difficult for me to share the sort of intellectual life that I had hoped for in a wife and this sometimes led to frustration with the shallowness of our companionship. We were still able to enjoy superficial activities together and I found pleasure in the domestic aspects of our daily life but emotionally I began to have difficulty with our inability to share things at a deeper level. Ann seemed not to be aware of this initially, probably because knowing that I was responsible for the situation I didn't want to hurt her and took care to hide my feelings. However, after a few months I did try to discuss things with her but this proved painful for both of us. Unfortunately at the same time she suffered a miscarriage that caused her great sadness and disappointment. Nevertheless, although I knew she was longing to start a family, I thought it wise to defer this until we could be more sure of our future. We both worked hard at this and over the next two years I could not but appreciate her kindness, loyalty and generous nature. She also came to understand me better, and although there were still occasional problems, it became clear we should stay together. Soon after reaching this conclusion Ann became pregnant with Katharine, the first of our four children, who all brought great joy to our lives and gave Ann the opportunity of fulfilling herself through motherhood. I became ever more immersed in my work, as a result of which I was frequently reminded of Yeats' couplet:

"The intellect of Man is forced to choose
Perfection of the work or of the life."

Anatomy Demonstrator
Once I had started in the Anatomy Department my relationship with Professor Warwick, though never cordial, improved. I was lucky to have Chris Adams and Richard Watson as the other two demonstrators as we got on well together and were able to learn from each other. Also having to teach anatomy to the students proved, as anticipated, the best way of mastering the subject in all its detail. There was also a lot of physiology and pathology to learn and I deferred taking the exam until February 1965 by which time I felt I had a good chance of passing. I recognised, however,

the uncertainty of this as the success rate of the Primary FRCS at that time was less than 20%. In the event, the papers and *vivas* went well and I was delighted to see my name amongst the successful candidates when the list was published in the College.

In early April Ann and I took our first proper holiday. We decided to explore the Lakes in Northern Italy and set off in my elderly Volkswagen, through France and Switzerland and then into Italy via the railway tunnel near Sion as the Simplon Pass was still closed by snow. The change in climate and scenery on the southern side of the Alps was dramatic, with welcome evidence of spring in the air. We spent two days in a small village near Lake Orta and then made our way East to Venice via Lakes Maggiore, Como, Lugano and Garda. Being so early in the season the locals seemed pleased to see us and we never had difficulty with securing accommodation. In Venice we stayed three days and then headed north out of Italy into Austria where we travelled via Salzburg to Berchtesgarten. There we spent the night before leaving the next morning in a blizzard for Munich and thence home. It was good to get away from London and work, the two weeks passed quickly and helped to resolve some of the difficulties Ann and I had been experiencing during the preceding year.

Junior Surgical Registrar at Guy's

Having passed the Primary Fellowship I now needed to get the necessary general surgical experience before I could sit the Final examination. To this end I was pleased to get one of the coveted appointments of Junior Surgical Registrar at Guy's. This did not start until October and I filled in the intervening time with locum posts; first as surgical SHO at Torquay and then with six weeks as Resident Surgical Officer (RSO) at the National Heart Hospital in London. I obtained the latter through the good offices of Donald Ross who, following his appointment at Guy's, had been invited to join the staff of the Heart Hospital. Cardiac surgery had started relatively late there, with Sir Thomas Holmes-Sellors being appointed first and then Donald Ross a few years later; and it was he who was largely responsible for its pre-eminent reputation in later years. Holmes-Sellors, or "Uncle Tom" as he was affectionately known by his juniors, was of the same generation as Brock, but of very different temperament. Ever courteous in the operating room, he was a fine craftsman and never blamed anyone else if things went wrong. He had done the first operation for the relief of pulmonary stenosis, but Brock followed quickly and got into print before him. Like Brock, he also later became President of the Royal College of Surgeons (1969-1972) and it was a great opportunity to work for him during this short period.

I started my Junior Registrarship at Guy's full of enthusiasm. The appointment was for a year and I was attached to the Glover-Beard Firm. Glover, the senior surgeon, had made his reputation through operating on varicose veins and was a good all round general surgeon. Beard was recently appointed to the consultant staff and was known to be a good technical surgeon. This was true, but he was at the stage when he liked to do the bulk of the operating himself and it was rare that he took the trouble to supervise one of his assistants with a case. So in some ways I found him disappointing to work for and when, after six months, the job of Resident Surgical Officer at the Bolingbroke Hospital in Wandsworth became vacant, I applied for this and was very pleased to get it.

Resident Surgical Officer at the Bolingbroke and London Chest Hospitals

The attraction of the Bolingbroke was that I would once again be working for Rex Lawrie. It was a small but busy hospital and the RSO was responsible for all the surgical patients, which apart from general surgery included urology and gynaecology. The visiting consultant staff were all eminent surgeons at London teaching hospitals. Besides Rex Lawrie, these included John Pullen, a general surgeon from St Thomas's Hospital, Peter Phillips, a urologist from Charing Cross, and George Pinker from St Mary's. He later became Obstetrician to the Royal Household and was then President of the Royal College of Obstetricians and Gynaecologists at the same time as I was President of the Royal College of Surgeons. Except for Mr Pullen they were all meticulous about fulfilling their duties at the Bolingbroke and I was soon embarked on a steep learning curve. Rex Lawrie was particularly helpful and I enjoyed the responsibility of being in charge when there were no consultants present, knowing that I could always call on him for advice and support if necessary. The on-call duties were onerous and comprised alternate nights with the RSO of Putney hospital, providing emergency cover for our respective hospitals. It was all excellent experience and by the end of a year I felt I had acquired enough knowledge to take the FRCS exam and get on with my cardiothoracic training. So in April 1967 I obtained a job as RSO at the London Chest Hospital and at the same time presented myself to the examiners. All went well during the papers and vivas except for the last one in operative surgery. There I encountered a most unsympathetic examiner who, having discovered I was weak in one particular operation, used up all the available time in concentrating on it. I duly failed. However, knowing that I needed to possess an FRCS diploma before being able to secure future good training posts, I went to Edinburgh two weeks later to sit their exam and came away with an FRCS. Ed. Six months later I re-sat the English exam and thankfully was more successful on that occasion.

My time at the London Chest Hospital provided me with a lot of good experience in Thoracic Surgery. Much of this was for cancer of the lung, which was only too common at the time and I found it distressing that so many of the cases were incurable, the cancer having spread beyond the confines of the lung. One of my consultants had the habit of breezily reassuring such patients on the ward round after the operation that "all had gone well". I was then placed in a difficult position when the patient and his or her relatives would subsequently want to know in more detail what had been found and what had been done. I felt sufficiently strongly about this that when I returned to the London Chest Hospital as a senior registrar eighteen months later I wrote a letter to *The Times*, which to my surprise was published. It contained the following:

"If asked, most members of the medical profession would probably express the wish to be told simply and truthfully when their own time came. Why therefore should our patients be denied the same right? I agree that each case should be judged on its merits and that there will undoubtedly be some who ought not to be told until near the end. However, it is my firm impression that in hospital practice too many are not told who ought to be and that the deception this involves, though perhaps well-meaning, is not in the true interest of our patients as human beings."

The Brompton, London Chest and National Heart Hospitals
Although my time at the London Chest was mostly well spent, it was my next job that proved so important in the context of further training. This was the sought after post as registrar to Mr Matt Paneth at the Brompton Hospital. He was the charismatic youngest consultant at the hospital and was recognised for providing his trainees with excellent experience. He was also known to demand a lot from them, as evidenced when he said to me after the interviews: "Well English, I don't like anyone other than my registrar looking after my patients. So you will be on call for the next year. If you need a night or a weekend off, let me know and I will consider standing in for you." And this is the way it turned out to be. I

was kept immensely busy, with the help of one RSO and an occasional visiting Fellow attached to his Firm. It was a long journey in the rush-hour from Blackheath to South Kensington, so I used to leave early after a large breakfast, which would keep me going for most of the day, and return home late, but only then if I was satisfied with the condition of my patients. Otherwise I would remain overnight in one of the rooms reserved for resident staff. The residents were well looked after at the Brompton. Dinner was a relatively formal affair and served promptly at seven minutes past seven in the teak-lined boardroom. Unusually, a thoughtful benefactor had seen fit to provide a small endowment that for many years allowed each resident to have a free bottle of beer with their meal. To make my journeys from Blackheath more pleasurable I brought a 1958 Porsche 356B, which turned out to be quite the nicest car to drive that I have ever had. Matt Paneth had a brand new Porsche and approved of my choice.

One of the operations that he had become well known for was emergency pulmonary embolectomy. This comprised the urgent removal of clots arising from the legs or pelvic veins and then blocking the circulation of blood through the lungs. These patients were usually in a parlous condition, the diagnosis often having been confused with a heart attack, and speed was of the utmost importance. Because of Paneth's interest in the condition, the Brompton had become the referral centre for London and most of the surrounding counties. It was his registrar who usually took the first call and who then had to effect the urgent transfer of the patient and arrange for X-ray facilities and a staffed operating room to be immediately available, whatever the hour of day or night. The operation itself was dramatic and indeed life saving. It comprised rapidly placing the patient on the heart-lung machine and then extracting the clots from the pulmonary arteries. Having done so, the circulation immediately improved and postoperative recovery was usually smooth.

Matt Paneth was a hard taskmaster but he also drove himself very hard and once I had gained his confidence we developed a good relationship. He had been trained by Brock and like him was a fine clinician and I learned a great deal during my time with him. He was also a supportive mentor and having discussed the possibilities of what I should do after my appointment came to an end in September 1968 he suggested that I was ready to apply for the senior registrar rotation between the Brompton, National Heart and London Chest Hospitals. He also offered to write to Albert Starr in Portland, Oregon, to recommend me for a clinical Fellowship for the year

1969. However, shortly before doing so I attended a lecture by John Kirklin who was visiting the Hammersmith hospital, and was so impressed that I said I would rather spend a year with him in Birmingham, Alabama, where he had recently moved from the Mayo Clinic. Matt therefore kindly wrote to Kirklin and I was then very pleased to be offered a research Fellowship for the year starting 1st January. The interviews for two senior registrar appointments were held in July and my good friend Christopher Lincoln and I were the successful candidates. This was a great relief as it meant for the first time that I had more or less security of tenure until becoming a consultant. It was agreed that I would spend the last three months of the year as senior registrar at the London Chest Hospital and then be allowed to take up my research Fellowship in America before returning to the rotation at the Brompton and National Heart hospitals. The three months at the London Chest passed rapidly and are remembered only for working for the most irascible surgeon I had ever encountered.

Research Fellow at Birmingham, Alabama

Our first son, Arthur, had been born in August 1968 so we went to Alabama with a young family. With no on-call duties and the more relaxed lifestyle of a research Fellow I looked forward to seeing more of Ann and the children than had been possible during the preceding two years. On arrival in Birmingham we found furnished accommodation in an apartment block close to the hospital for the first six months and then rented a pleasant old house with a large garden at 117 West Glenwood Drive, in the suburb of Homewood. I had an introduction to a bank manager through a contact in South Africa and this led to us meeting Vann and Ann Henagan from whom we bought their 4-year old Chevrolet. This served us well in our travels throughout the Southern States during the next year and the Henagans also became and remain good friends. It was an interesting time to be in the South, both socially and politically. Martin Luther King had been assassinated the previous year and the Civil Rights campaign was gathering momentum. This was being resisted by Governor George Wallace and his conservative supporters and in many respects the situation reminded me of what was going on in South Africa. The continuing Vietnam War was also the source of much controversy, with the Southerners being inherently patriotic and yet confused as to whether American troops should really be there. During the year we made many good friends amongst them and I enjoyed having a more normal family life with the luxury of seeing Ann and the children both at breakfast and in the evenings.

Professionally, it also turned out to be amongst the most interesting and important of my years of training. Problems with lung function after open-heart surgery were still common at the time and my research, which had been suggested by Kirklin, was centred around trying to define what factors were involved in this. Bob Karp, who had just been appointed Assistant Professor of Surgery, helped me with theoretical aspects of the project and for the animal experiments I had the expert technical assistance of Stan Digerness. This kept me occupied me in laboratory work throughout the year, but I didn't want to leave without being exposed to what was going on in the operating theatre. So I designed a short research project studying fluctuations of colloid osmotic pressure during cardiopulmonary bypass, which required me to be in theatre for the duration of an operation. This provided the opportunity of seeing Dr Kirklin at work, as well as some of his talented younger colleagues. As mentioned, he had been involved in open-heart surgery since its very inception and was becoming one of the most influential cardiac surgeons of his generation. I had become used to the fact that patients occasionally died after cardiac surgery but Kirklin had a passion to, as he put it, " reduce operative mortality to zero" and in this his logic was impeccable. He would say that if one always operated on the basis of the right diagnosis, and if the operation was performed correctly with meticulous attention to detail so that the patient's circulatory state was always better at the end of the operation than before you started, and that the patient was looked after correctly during the recovery period, one should never have a death. Inevitably, of course deaths still did occur even in his unit. But each one would provide the basis for a careful analysis of every step in the procedure until some error in judgement or execution could be defined, which had led to the unfortunate outcome. The educational value of this process, which was shared with the whole team, and the careful statistical analysis of the incremental risk factors associated with individual operations, provided an invaluable discipline on which to base future practice. Indeed, it was largely this experience which, as I shall describe later, stimulated me to establish the UK Cardiac Surgical Register.

During the year in Alabama Ann became pregnant with our third child and as the baby was due at the end of December she returned to England in mid-November with Katharine and Arthur while I finished writing up my research. They stayed initially with our friends, Des and Judy Carroll and then moved back into 'The Quantocks' where I joined them in time for Mary's birth on 1st January. Soon after Ann returned home with Mary I realised that we had outgrown our existing accommodation and began to look for a house to buy. While engaged in this I was fortunate to find one across the Heath in Pond Road that was being offered for sale by a Commander Worth. It was a large Victorian house with a big garden adjoining Blackheath village and close to the railway station. Our negotiations usually took place over a glass of whisky and whenever I tried to make an offer he seemed embarrassed and brought up something else before offering me another drink, so that it took some time to clinch the deal. Having done so, the 'Red Cottage' provided a fine home for us until we moved to Cambridge three years later.

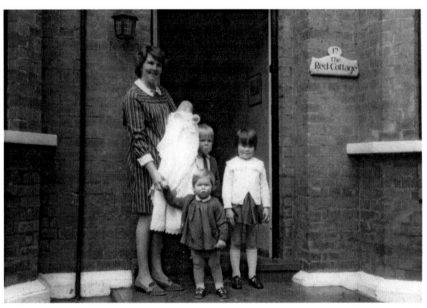

At the "Red Cottage" – William's Christening

On my return to England I was scheduled to spend the next year at the Brompton as senior registrar to Mr Cleland and Stuart Lennox. Although I had seen a lot I was still relatively inexperienced in personal operative surgery and it soon became clear that more was expected of me than I felt comfortable with. Bill Cleland also had a busy practice at the Hammersmith hospital and it was not unusual to receive a phone call from him and be asked to carry on with his afternoon list because he was held up. It wasn't that I didn't know what needed doing but simply that I was aware of my technical shortcomings and took longer over the cases than I would have liked. However, with the passage of time my technique improved and I became adjusted to the responsibility, so that by the end of the year I was able to enjoy the satisfaction of completing quite complex operations on my own and in good time.

This served me in good stead when I transferred to the National Heart Hospital at the beginning of 1971. There I spent the first six months with Donald Ross and the last six with his namesake, Keith Ross. Donald was present for the first two weeks after my arrival and then went abroad for the next fortnight. It was the custom for the senior registrar to operate on his patients while he was away and I chose to select from his waiting list the oldest patients I could find, believing that if any of the patients died it would be better if they were old rather than young. Thankfully all survived and my choice seemed to impress Donald as he indicated this was not what usually happened when he was away. I had great pleasure working with him, trying to incorporate his superb technical skills, which I could never satisfactorily match. He was also good to me treating me both as professional colleague and friend as, for example, when William was born in April, he sent his secretary Margaret Alabaster to Marylebone High Street to buy the largest and most expensive cigar she could find for the proud father.

Keith Ross was also a good surgeon but I suspect he felt at somewhat of a disadvantage, believing that his trainees might compare his technical skills unfavourably with those of Donald's. For most of us this was not the case and again I had an enjoyable and productive relationship with him during my last six months at the National Heart Hospital. An interesting event happened halfway through this period. A consultant post came up unexpectedly in Southampton as a result of the anaesthetists refusing to work for the senior surgeon because of his lack of discipline with regard to his theatre duties. I knew the two cardiologists in the Unit and having looked into what the job offered was encouraged by one of them to apply. Having done so, Keith told me that he had heard about the job and offered to act as one of my referees. I thanked him but pointed out that I had already asked Donald Ross, Matt Paneth and John Kirklin to act in that capacity. Shortly after this conversation Keith left for an extended visit to New Zealand. I was subsequently short-listed for interview, which was to be preceded by a less formal "trial by sherry" the night before the main interviews, which would be attended by all the consultant staff from the Unit and the four short-listed candidates. By now I was keen to get the job and decided to prepare for the interviews by two days walking in the Black Mountains in Wales before driving to Southampton. To my dismay I was caught in a traffic jam on the way there and arrived 15 minutes after the informal interviews had started. As I came in I saw Keith Ross across the room and gave him a smile, believing that he must be present as the Royal College's assessor. However, he looked embarrassed and within a short time I realised that he was also a candidate for the job! He explained immediately afterwards that while in New Zealand he began to think how much happier he would be in Southampton than in London and had therefore put in a late application. Understandably the opportunity of having an established consultant to rebuild confidence in the Unit was not to be missed and he was duly appointed. I gathered later that I was the 'runner-up' and looking back on it now I am grateful for Keith's unexpected intervention, as although I am sure I would have been happy in Southampton, I believe I was able to achieve more at Papworth.

The final year of my senior registrarship was back at the Brompton, this time working for both Mr Oswald Tubbs, the senior surgeon, and Matt Paneth. 'Os' was in the last year of his career and was clearly finding operating a strain. He was also painfully slow and querulous and it was not much fun assisting him. However, my work with Matt made up for this and as the year proceeded I felt increasingly ready to take on the role of independent practice.

Chapter 5.
Papworth Hospital and Heart Transplantation

One day towards the end of 1972 I was operating with Matt Paneth, when he turned to the anaesthetist and asked, "Do you think English would get on with Milstein". I enquired who Milstein was and was told that he was a surgeon working in a small hospital called Papworth in the Cambridgeshire Fens and that he was looking for a locum for three months. Matt suggested that I should investigate and so I went to Papworth, liked what I saw and accepted the job, leaving Ann and our four young children in Blackheath.

By the time the three months had passed I had got to know and admire Ben Milstein. He also wanted me to stay and I liked his proposal that we should work together as a team, sharing facilities and junior staff and be willing to learn from each other; a remarkable attitude coming from a forceful character 15 years my senior. The locum post had arisen as a result of Ben's senior colleague, Chris Parish, having been appointed Postgraduate Dean for the East Anglian Region. So when the substantive post came up in February 1973 I applied and was pleased to be appointed Consultant Cardiothoracic Surgeon to Papworth and Addenbrooke's Hospital in Cambridge. My job description, as I recall, was admirably brief and was simply "to provide a cardiothoracic surgical service to the patients of East Anglia." Rather different from what is contained in current contracts!

In May 1973 I obtained two weeks study leave to visit the Mayo Clinic in Rochester and Stanford University in California. During this trip I was accompanied by my good friend Christopher Lincoln who had just been appointed consultant to the Brompton Hospital in London where we had both trained. I particularly wanted to visit Stanford in order to see a friend Philip Caves who, after spending a year in the laboratory, had so impressed Dr Shumway that he had been made Chief Resident and given the singular honour of being put in charge of the transplant programme. Philip and I had become firm friends whilst training at the Brompton, when he was a registrar and I senior registrar. And like all who knew him I had been impressed by his extraordinary energy and ability – a truly driven person who sadly died from a heart attack at the early age of 38 by which time he had progressed to Professor of Cardiac Surgery in Glasgow.

Whilst staying with Philip in Stanford I was interested to see patients who were doing well after heart transplantation and I became inspired by his enthusiasm for its future. Although Barnard had done the first heart transplant, Shumway and his colleague Richard Lower had done nearly all the early important experimental work, refining the surgical technique and investigating the phenomenon of rejection after transplantation and how this might be modified. So their disappointment was great when Barnard achieved primacy by doing the first case. As mentioned, I had spent a week in 1963 observing Barnard's work in Cape Town and had come away unimpressed by his technical skills and behaviour in the operating theatre, although I had to recognise his good results which derived from an obsessive attention to detail. So like many others, I was surprised to hear of his first two transplants on 3rd December 1967 and 2nd January 1968. Shumway followed with his first on 6th January and soon cardiac surgeons all over the world were attempting to transplant hearts, usually with poor results. Indeed of the 166 patients who received hearts during 1968, 1969 and 1970 only just over half lived for more than a month and 11% more than two years. Amongst these were three patients transplanted by my mentor Donald Ross, but in keeping with results elsewhere in the world they only survived for short periods (45, 2 and 107 days). So in January 1973, the Chief Medical Officer for Health, Sir George Godber, declared what amounted to a moratorium on further attempts at heart transplantation in Britain.

During these early years Norman Shumway had pressed on with a careful and responsible programme at Stanford and by the time of my visit was getting encouraging results. Much of the improvement was due to the clinical introduction of biopsy of the heart that allowed acute rejection to be detected earlier and hence treated more effectively than had previously been possible. This technique had been developed in the laboratory by

Philip Caves and involved passing a catheter into the heart to take small fragments of tissue that could then be examined under the microscope for signs of rejection. The technique also proved valuable in monitoring the response to augmented treatment for rejection so that this did not need to be unduly prolonged with the ensuing danger of infection.

In any event, I left Stanford impressed by what had been achieved during the preceding five years, and felt that it was time for England to have at least one centre where heart transplantation was being pursued. I should add that at this time I was unaware of the moratorium that Godber placed on further transplant activity earlier that year. So on return to Papworth I discussed the matter with Ben Milstein. Ben, whilst not wishing to be personally involved, was most supportive and remained so during the trials and tribulations which followed. He suggested that I take the matter up with the Professor of Surgery in Cambridge, Roy Calne, who had already established kidney and liver transplantation in Cambridge. This I did and Roy responded enthusiastically. Clearly it was necessary to seek the support of colleagues at both Papworth and Addenbrooke's and the first formal meeting to explore this took place in October 1973. It was apparent from the start that neither of the two cardiologists at Papworth wished to be involved. Hugh Fleming was neutral in his stance whereas David Evans expressed strong opposition based on clinical, ethical and religious grounds. Subsequently, during all the years that followed, he remained highly critical of the work and could never accept the diagnosis of brain death, thereby leading him to accuse me on a number of occasions of removing hearts from people who were still alive.

However, at that initial meeting agreement was reached, with David Evans dissenting, that we would work towards establishing heart transplantation at Cambridge. Because of Roy's transplant programme donor organs became available at Addenbrooke's and it was envisaged that the operation and early postoperative care would take place in his Department of Surgery. As a preliminary, it was agreed that I should join Roy's experimental programme and that we would also establish familiarity with routine cardiac surgery at Addenbrooke's. To this end, approval needed to be obtained from the relevant medical committees at Addenbrooke's and for their operating theatre staff to get experience with cardiac surgical procedures at Papworth.

This all took some time during which it became clear to me that some service departments at Addenbrooke's were concerned by the prospect of adding heart transplantation to the existing demand on resources made by the liver and kidney transplant programmes. However, permission was eventually, albeit somewhat reluctantly given, with the proviso that we should report back to the Hospital Medical Committee before actually proceeding to transplantation. So having trained the necessary Intensive Care, theatre staff and heart-lung machine technicians at Addenbrooke's we did a series of open-heart operations there in the autumn of 1974, with Professor Calne and his Senior Registrar assisting me and with the anaesthetists from Papworth. These were successful and by completion we felt that the experience gained indicated that the facility for performing open-heart surgery at Addenbrooke's, on which transplantation depended, was now established.

The experimental work also went well and we began to get more regular survivors after transplanting hearts into pigs. Then in March 1976 the Professor of Medicine, Ivor Mills, who was well known for his scepticism as to the value of cardiac surgery, surprisingly referred me a patient for consideration of transplantation. I was due to leave for a meeting in Hong Kong in a few days but before doing so I made a careful assessment of the patient who was 59 years old and had an advanced cardiomyopathy (muscle disease of the heart). He had suffered severe loss of weight due to long-standing heart failure with incipient gangrene of his toes and I considered him too old and too sick to be suitable for transplantation. (At that time, in keeping with Stanford's protocol we had decided on an upper age limit for potential recipients of 50 years). However, I asked Hugh Fleming to see the patient and he concurred with my decision. I then wrote to Roy Calne, with a copy to Ivor Mills, providing them with a full report of my assessment and left for Hong Kong. On my return ten days later I was dismayed to learn that during my absence Roy had unilaterally decided to proceed with an immediate transplant if a donor could be found. In the event one was not forthcoming and the patient died a few days before I got back. However, the reaction to Roy's decision at Addenbrooke's was intense, and we were forcefully reminded of our agreement to seek approval from the Medical Committee before embarking on human heart transplantation.

This episode caused me to question Roy's judgement and also to recognise the difficulties associated with establishing the work at Addenbrooke's, where many of the medical staff seemed to be opposed to it. So I began to believe that the right place for the programme had to be Papworth

Hospital. As a cardiac surgical procedure it was logical that the operation should be done by cardiac surgeons, assisted by anaesthetists and nursing staff who were familiar with dealing with very sick cardiac patients on a daily basis and with dedicated operating theatre and intensive care facilities on site. I also considered the general ambience of Papworth more suitable for potentially long-stay transplant patients and their families than that of Addenbrooke's. At a meeting after my return from Hong Kong I expressed these views to Roy, who not surprisingly found them difficult to accept. By this time he had an international reputation as a transplant surgeon and I was virtually unknown. However, I remained convinced that my decision was the best way forward and no agreement was reached.

In April we were asked to meet Dr Robertson, the Cambridge Area Medical Officer, to let him know what our plans were and in July he convened a more formal meeting with wide representation from Papworth and Addenbrooke's. Again no decisions were made apart from seeking further information on the likely demand on resources as well as an appreciation of cost effectiveness and how best to select patients. In October of the same year a report was published by the Conference of UK Medical Royal Colleges and their Faculties, clearly defining the clinical criteria for diagnosing brain death. This was a most important event as, although primarily directed at the management of patients with severe brain damage in Intensive Care Units, the report also had implications for procuring suitable hearts for transplantation. The Chief Medical Officer alluded to this in a letter distributed to all hospital doctors in which he wrote:

"The conclusion that respiration (breathing) and a beating heart are being maintained solely by mechanical means and that brain death has occurred is reached entirely independently of any transplant consideration. However, once the diagnosis of death has been made the actual moment at which a respirator is switched off may be influenced by the need to maintain the kidneys or other organs in the best possible condition before they are removed for an eventual transplant."

Until this time kidneys were removed from donors whose hearts had stopped and who had been without a circulation for some time. If the kidney did not work immediately after transplantation, the patient could be maintained on dialysis until recovery took place. No such support was available for heart patients beyond an hour or two on a heart-lung machine. So being able to remove a heart from a brain-dead donor in whom the circulation was still intact meant that good quality hearts could be obtained for transplantation and this was a great step forward for us.

Around the same time as the report on Brain Death was published I submitted a grant application to the Regional Health Authority to pursue my own research programme at Huntingdon Research Centre. This is a private institution that later attracted much attention from the animal rights activists, who thankfully never succeeded in their objective of closing it down. My grant was approved and in January 1977 I embarked on a two-year project aimed at finding the best way of preserving and storing donor hearts so that they could be transplanted safely after having been procured at distant hospitals and then transported to Papworth. Using pigs as the experimental animal we devised a technique of perfusing the intact heart with chemicals to arrest it and then cooling it to 4°C, after which it was stored in a similar solution and transported in a simple coolbox. In this way we showed that the heart was not damaged by temporary lack of oxygen, and that its energy supplies could be conserved for periods of four to six hours. I judged this would be long enough for us to contemplate transporting donor hearts from anywhere in the United Kingdom to Papworth, with sufficient confidence that they would perform well after transplantation.

In February 1977 there was some movement in the attitude of the Department of Health towards heart transplantation in that a Transplant Advisory Panel, chaired by the Chief Medical Officer, defined the criteria that would have to be met by any centre wishing to embark on heart transplants. These included reference to having adequate support services in pathology, immunology, microbiology and radiology and the ability to maintain both a transplant programme and the regular cardiac work. It also declared that preferably kidney transplantation should be based at the same centre. The latter, while not at Papworth, was taking place nearby in Cambridge and I did not regard this as an absolute contra-indication.

Also of importance during this same year was the appointment of Michael Petch as third consultant cardiologist to Papworth and Addenbrooke's. I had known Michael since 1971 when we were both working at the National Heart Hospital and was delighted when he agreed to provide cardiological support to the transplant programme and to share the responsibility of selecting potential recipients for transplantation. Our agreement was that we would review referrals independently and only accept a patient if we both agreed that transplantation was indicated. I should add that his participation came despite strong pressure from David Evans not to become involved.

By January 1978 we had been referred two patients from outside the East Anglian Region whom we considered suitable for transplantation. I then met with the Chairman, Mrs Pauline Burnett, and officers of the Area Health Authority responsible for Papworth and Addenbrooke's hospitals, and told them of our plans for starting a heart transplant programme at Papworth. I also shared with them the protocols I had prepared for the meeting of the Transplant Advisory Panel (TAP) scheduled for the following month.

Pauline Burnett was gratifyingly sympathetic to our cause and agreed to await the response from the TAP. At my request, she also agreed that our plans should remain confidential and not be brought to the full membership of the Authority, at least for the time being, as I did not want any unwelcome publicity before we had done the first case.

The Transplant Advisory Panel met on 3rd February. I had prepared a document entitled "Clinical Cardiac Transplantation in Cambridge" which I forwarded to the Panel before the meeting. This outlined a programme with the donor operation being done at Addenbrooke's and the assessment, recipient operation and postoperative management taking place at Papworth. This did not find favour with Roy Calne, who was a member of the TAP, and who still wanted both operations to be done in his department at Addenbrooke's. However, I was relieved that he did not express these views to the committee.

After a full discussion the Advisory panel agreed that I had made a good case for a clinical programme of cardiac transplantation but that no central funding should be made available for such a programme. They also indicated that they would not approve of any "one-off operations" thereby virtually blocking further progress. However, by now I had devoted so much time trying to establish a heart transplant programme, during which I had become convinced that we ought to be able to replicate the good results coming from Stanford, that I decided to carry on. So I went back to Mrs. Burnett and the officers of the Health Authority and, after further discussions, they tacitly and courageously agreed that they would support my using our existing facilities at Papworth for two cases but that thereafter funding for a continuing programme would have to be found from elsewhere. And it was on this basis that we proceeded.

The rest of 1978 was a lean and frustrating year as we were unable to secure any donor hearts. Roy remained unhelpful and when I met the senior neurosurgeon at Addenbrooke's, Walpole Lewin, he was unwilling to give this any priority. I visited four other Neurosurgical Units in London, informing them of our needs and asking for help, but despite varying degrees of offers of support, nothing was forthcoming. Amongst renal transplant surgeons that I knew, Michael Bewick and Chris Rudge in London declared their willingness to help but the result was the same. I also made a further visit to Stanford following which I received a most helpful letter from Norman Shumway encouraging me to persist with our attempts to establish heart transplantation in England. By this time my friend Philip Caves had returned from Stanford, first to Edinburgh and then to a Chair in Cardiac Surgery at Glasgow. There he was so busy dealing with routine adult and paediatric heart surgery that he had to put plans for cardiac transplantation temporarily on hold. Sadly, his tragic early death meant that he never achieved this.

In October I had another meeting with Roy Calne but he remained adamant that there could be no further collaboration as long as the transplants were to be done at Papworth. Another issue between us at this time was his desire to use the new drug cyclosporine as the sole immunosuppressive agent as he had started doing with kidney transplantation earlier in the year. However, I was keen to continue with the Stanford protocol (using azathioprine and steroids) as I felt not enough was yet known about the potential side-effects of cyclosporine. In this my decision was vindicated, as Roy's early experience with cyclosporine on its own was associated with a high incidence of kidney toxicity and malignant tumours, and it was left to Tom Starzl in America to show that it needed to be combined with steroids to provide a safer and more effective anti-rejection regime.

However, whereas 1978 had been a disappointing year, that all changed in 1979. It started with an excellent article in the British Medical Journal from Dr Shumway's group, reviewing experience with their first 150 patients of whom 70% survived one year with a 5% per annum mortality thereafter. This was amongst patients who were not expected to live on average more than six months. Their paper was accompanied by a leading article, which was cautiously supportive of heart transplantation being pursued in other centres. At this time, the only active units other than Stanford were Barnard's in Cape Town, Richard Lower's in Richmond, Virginia, and Christian Cabrol's in Paris.

On 14th January, the day after the publication of this article, and with Professor Calne out of town, his senior registrar, Paul McMaster, phoned me in the afternoon to say that he had received permission for both heart and kidneys to be used from a donor in Addenbrooke's. This was the breakthrough we had been waiting for. The size of the heart and blood group were suitable for one of our potential recipients, a 44 year old bachelor, Charles McHugh, who had by then spent a prolonged time in Papworth with advanced heart disease and who was now seriously ill. Having obtained his agreement and spoken to his sister who was a nursing sister in Surrey, we made plans to go ahead with the operation that evening. I had previously decided that I should do both the donor and the transplant operation as I felt the responsibility of assessing the donor and the suitability of the heart prior to its removal should be mine. So I went to Addenbrooke's to do the donor operation with the assistance of Paul McMaster, whilst I left my experienced senior registrar, David Cooper, at Papworth to prepare McHugh for the transplant and start opening his chest once I gave word that the donor heart had been removed and was in good condition. Just as I had completed this I was phoned by Don Bethune our anaesthetist at Papworth, to say that a short time previously McHugh's heart had stopped. He had been rapidly resuscitated and after opening his chest David Cooper had placed him on the support of the heart-lung machine, thereby providing a secure circulation to his vital organs. However, Don went on to say that although the situation was now stable, he could not be sure whether McHugh might have suffered a degree of brain damage during the relatively brief period of cardiac arrest, although on balance he thought probably not.

This presented me with a very difficult decision but I decided to go ahead with the transplant on the basis of Don's opinion and in the knowledge that McHugh would now certainly not survive without a transplant. So I returned rapidly to Papworth and, having excised his heart, proceeded with the transplant. The operation went smoothly and it was then that I realised how valuable the many pig heart transplants had been that David and I and the rest of the team had done at Huntingdon Research Centre.

Once the operation was complete the donor heart worked beautifully and there was a sense of great elation amongst all those in the operating room.

McHugh was returned to the Intensive Care Unit soon after midnight and I then spoke to his sister who by now had arrived at Papworth. I told her of what had happened and of our concern that there was a possibility that he might have suffered some brain damage. She was very understanding and expressed relief that he should have at least been given the chance of life.

The next morning all seemed to be well. The new heart continued to work perfectly and his kidneys and other organs were functioning satisfactorily. He was still on the ventilator so it was too early to assess his brain function. News of the transplant was broken that morning by John Edwards, the Regional Press Officer, with whom we had worked closely. Initially, when planning how to handle the media, he had wanted to be more forthcoming than I was prepared to allow. I was very conscious of the adverse impact on public and professional opinion that had occurred as a result of the way the press and television had been handled after Donald Ross's transplant operations and was determined that we should do things better. We therefore decided that John Edwards should be the sole mouthpiece for Papworth; that personalities should be kept to a minimum, and that reference should generally be made simply to the "Papworth Team". He explained that it would be impossible not to refer to me as the leader of the team but that he would keep press conferences etc to an absolute minimum. The first Press Conference after McHugh's operation did in fact take place two days later. This was held at Addenbrooke's attended by Michael Petch, Dr Donald Robertson (Area Medical Officer) and me. Roy Calne was invited but declined to be present. The degree of interest was by then intense and it was painful to have to express my concern that the patient, who was doing well in every other respect, had not yet recovered normal brain function. It was gratifying, however, to receive a personal note from the Chief Medical Officer, Sir Henry Yellowlees, dated 26th January saying: "May I thank you for the discretion you have shown in your approach to the present case and congratulate you on the way in which you have handled the publicity. I hope the clinical position is improving. An official invitation to the Transplant Advisory Panel on February 9th is enclosed – I hope you will come."

In the event McHugh never did recover normal brain function and as this entailed keeping him on a ventilator for prolonged periods he inevitably developed a fatal lung infection and died 17 days after his transplant. Naturally this came as a huge disappointment to all of us associated with the project but, having seen the dramatic effect of providing a patient in terminal heart failure with a normal functioning heart, I was determined to carry on and not be deterred by this unfortunate failure of our first case.

I had a difficult meeting with Roy Calne five days later. He was very critical of what had happened and, although unaware of all the facts, this did not deter him from declaring that I had set back cardiac transplantation in Britain by five years. I reiterated that I felt he could still have an important role and that our case would be stronger if his department in Cambridge were associated with the project but that I remained convinced the clinical work could only be done at Papworth. I also expressed my concern that if the current division between us became more widely known it would be bad for both our reputations and that our proposals would be less likely to get the approval of the Department of Health.

The Transplant Advisory Panel met on 9th February, ten days after McHugh's death. Failure of the operation had drawn criticism from all sorts of quarters, both lay and professional, and I was invited to attend to "tell members of the Panel about the case and inform them of our future plans." As anticipated, it proved a difficult meeting. Although there was support from some members, Roy declared "that until the problems posed by the separation of the cardiac facilities at Papworth Hospital from Addenbrooke's were overcome, Cambridge was unsuitable for setting up a cardiac transplant programme." The Chairman, Sir Henry Yellowlees, said that this was a problem for local resolution, and although the Panel was generally supportive of the concept of establishing and funding a programme, the Chief Medical Officer later reaffirmed that "Ministers did not consider that the diversion of resources to such a programme would be justified at this stage". All very depressing. However, a few days later I was gratified to receive an encouraging letter from Professor John Goodwin, a respected cardiologist, President of the Cardiac Society and a member of the TAP, in which he wrote: "of course transplantation must go on in Cambridge. It occurs to me that Papworth is the right place, and I do hope the Calne problem can be sorted out." In responding to him I concluded: "Certainly I can see no way that the work could be pursued anywhere other than where the cardiologists, cardiac surgeons and anaesthetists normally practise. In the meantime we shall carry on in the belief that we have tried to act responsibly and that the most effective answer to criticism would be the accomplishment of a few successful cases."

On 24th March 1979 I wrote again to Roy informing him that we had accepted another potential recipient and, recognising that he was going to be away for four weeks, asked whether he would be agreeable to Paul McMaster helping me secure the heart if a suitable donor became available in Addenbrooke's as I assumed no liver transplants would be done during his absence. He responded two days later that "he and his colleagues remained very worried at the effect that requesting for heart donation may have on our kidney donations and that therefore unless the relatives of a potential donor specifically request that the heart be used for transplantation, we should not be involved in trying to get hearts".

And so things remained in deadlock. Dr Robertson visited the Department of Health to try and find out on what basis the Department would or would not approve a programme. I also wrote to Sir John Butterfield, Regius Professor of Physic in Cambridge, to seek his good offices in asking Sir Henry Yellowlees to arrange for a few members of the TAP to make site visits to both Addenbrooke's and Papworth and then make a recommendation based on their findings as to where the work should be pursued. Sir John used his formidable diplomatic skills to try and mediate an agreement between Roy Calne and me. However, I remained insistent that the work could only be carried out at Papworth and although I agreed to Roy assisting with both donor and recipient operations and with advice on immunosuppression, his position became more entrenched and he established a policy that his team would not remove kidneys if I obtained permission for removal of the heart.

And then on 18th August Paul McMaster informed me that a donor was present in RAF Ely Hospital, whose parents had specifically asked that all possible organs should be used for transplantation. Roy was again out of town so this enabled us to go ahead, and Paul also secured the kidneys and pancreas for transplantation. Our recipient was Keith Castle, a 52-year-old builder from Wandsworth in London whom we had accepted after assessment some six weeks earlier. Both donor and recipient operations proceeded smoothly and it was a huge relief that his postoperative recovery was for the most part uncomplicated apart from one mild bout of rejection. Keith was not an ideal candidate in that he was a heavy smoker with a history of chronic duodenal ulcer and established peripheral vascular disease as well as his heart disease. But he had great humour and fortitude and in every other respect could not have been a better patient. He subsequently became the best possible advertisement for cardiac transplantation, except for his inability to give up smoking which I had tried hard to get him to stop but without success. A few months after his discharge from hospital we presented his case at Grand Surgical Rounds at Addenbrooke's to which Keith was invited. The lecture theatre was packed to overflowing and during the questions which followed, Dr Robertson who was an ardent Public Health and anti-smoking doctor, asked him rather pointedly if he was still smoking. Keith looked briefly at me and then replied "Certainly not." "Oh", said Dr Robertson, "but I heard you were." "No", replied Keith,

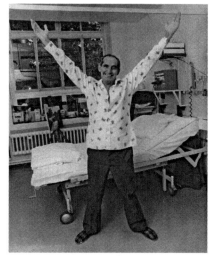

Keith Castle, before discharge following his transplant.

"Mr English told me not to." Quite a few of those present, including of course me, knew that this was not true but he was determined not to let the side down in front of such a large medical audience, for which of course I forgave him. Keith later became somewhat of a national figure as well as an icon for future heart transplant patients. His cockney wit, cheerfulness and enduring optimism, and his gratitude for the extra five and a half years of life granted him, which he put to such good effect, endeared him to everyone he met.

Soon after his operation I was able to announce that I had obtained funding from the National Heart Research Fund to cover the costs of the next six patients. This was in keeping with the original agreement that the Area Health Authority would only be responsible for funding the first two cases and helped to mollify some of the more critical members of the Authority. And then later in the year, due to the wise and persistent diplomacy of John Butterfield, agreement was reached as to how Roy Calne and I might collaborate in the future. In essence it was accepted that the clinical work could only be done at Papworth but that he would become involved with both donor and recipient operations. Also that he would advise on immunosuppression and that we would work towards introducing a cyclosporine-based regime in 6 to 18 months.

On the 22nd November we transplanted Andrew Barlow, a 29-year-old man with advanced coronary disease, with Roy assisting. The operation went smoothly and Andrew duly left hospital much improved and was soon leading a virtually normal life. That same month the Transplant Advisory Panel met again and having received cost estimates for a programme of eight transplants per year prepared by the Department using data from our first two cases which amounted to £17,300 per patient per first year, noted "that results at Papworth had shown that heart transplantation was a viable proposition with a potential future and confirmed their view that the hospital complied with the criteria for a planned programme of development". This opinion was then transmitted to the Secretary of State for Health for his approval and decision on funding.

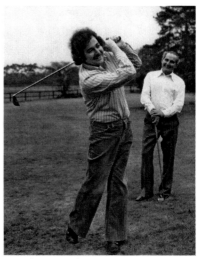

Andrew Barlow and Keith Castle playing golf.

On 10th December I wrote to the Chief Medical Officer asking for confirmation of official recognition and funding for Papworth. I also mentioned the need to control the development of cardiac transplantation in Britain as I had heard of four other centres that might be considering heart transplants. I suggested that all Cardiac Surgical Units should be sent an official memorandum advising them of the criteria set by the Transplant Advisory Panel before starting transplantation. I also pointed out that if our Unit were to be officially recognised by the Department of Health and was known to be receiving funding from the Department, it might be easier to dissuade other centres from starting at the present time, as it could be correctly stated that the Department was already supporting a pilot clinical programme at Papworth.

On 9th January (1980) I received a polite response from Sir Henry saying that he would let Regional and Area Medical Officers know the outcome of the discussion at the last TAP meeting, but that he would be misleading me if he held out hope that central NHS funds, additional to those managed by the Area Health Authority, could be found for a transplant programme at Papworth. Sir Henry also referred to the Cambridge Area Health Authority having initiated a study by the Department of Community Medicine to investigate the workings of the cardiological and surgical departments at Papworth and to estimate what impact a transplant programme would have on the hospital, and that until this had been completed "decisions about the next steps at Papworth were not possible". In the meantime, using funds from the National Heart Research Fund, we were able to appoint a laboratory technician in Clinical Immunology at Addenbrooke's and one in Biochemistry at Papworth, and do another successful transplant.

The report from the Department of Community Medicine was received by the Area Health Authority at their meeting on 12th February, having received input from various other Committees. The report concluded that "if adequate financial support is forthcoming, there is no reason why Papworth Hospital should not be capable of supporting a programme of cardiac transplantation, provided that the other services at the hospital are safeguarded", and its final sentence read, "indeed, the improved recruitment and morale generated by a transplant programme might be important factors in securing rapid implementation of other developments at the hospital". Having debated the matter, the Area Health Authority recommended to the Regional Health Authority and the Department of Health that a programme of heart transplants should be undertaken at Papworth Hospital on the understanding that the cost is not charged to the normal revenue funding of the Area Health Authority. Also that necessary provision is made to protect the normal working of the Regional Cardiothoracic Services and that this should continue to be monitored.

Later in February we did two more transplants and during the same month Magdi Yacoub did his first transplant at Harefield. When looking back on these first six crucial transplants the results were relatively gratifying in that two of them lived for more than eight years, one for five and a half years, and one for three years. To date the longest Papworth survivor, who was transplanted in September 1980, lived for 26 years. In any event five of our first six patients were alive when, on 13th March 1980, the Secretary of State for Social Services, Mr Patrick Jenkin, announced in Parliament that the Transplant Advisory Panel had accepted Papworth Hospital as suitable for a planned programme of heart transplantation. He confirmed that "Cambridgeshire Area Health Authority are satisfied, after a detailed study, that given improvements to the operating theatre and intensive care facilities at Papworth and appropriate financial support, a programme could be undertaken without detriment to other services". He then went on to announce that the Robinson Charitable Trust had donated £300,000 for heart transplant work at Papworth in 1981 and 1982, and that in the light of this donation he had agreed to make a special allocation of up to £100,000 to cover the capital cost of improving the operating theatres and intensive care unit; and also that he would be prepared to provide some additional revenue support during 1980 if this was necessary. This was all very encouraging but did not prevent one of my favourite journalists, Bernard Levin, commenting in "The Times" as follows:

" The fashion for heart transplants, like fashion in hemlines, will soon be forgotten and replaced by some other operation. The history of medicine is bestrewn with brief enthusiasms of no ultimate value to anybody except the doctors."

The story behind the Robinson donation is an interesting one. David Robinson was a local Cambridge millionaire who had already provided £17 million to found Robinson College. He was also a great recluse. Pauline Burnett, Chairman of the Area Health Authority, had suggested that I approach him for help with funding and I did so without much expectation of success and with great difficulty in getting the application to him. I heard nothing from him for several weeks and then, on returning home late one evening from work, I heard Katharine, then aged 13, saying on the telephone: "No, you cannot possibly speak to Daddy unless you tell me who you are". I took the phone and a voice said, "Is that you, Mr English?" and after confirming that it was, the voice said, "You are a very difficult man to get hold of, Mr English". On being told who I was speaking to, I could only reply, "But Mr Robinson, you are far more difficult to get hold of". There was a short chuckle from the other end and then an appointment was made to see him and his secretary, Miss Umney, at his hideaway in the Newmarket woods three days later. At that meeting the chemistry was right and before leaving he had agreed to support my application for £300,000 over the two years, 1981 and 1982.

In April 1980 I submitted a grant application to the British Heart Foundation for £60,000 per annum for five years towards funding a BHF Heart Transplant Research Group at Papworth, of which I would be the Honorary Director. This was approved in July and allowed the appointment of Richard Cory-Pearce (our then senior registrar) as Senior Research Fellow with honorary consultant status; as well as a Research Fellow in Immunology based at Addenbrooke's, a Senior Research Technician at Papworth and a Secretary.

In May, Ben Milstein and I wrote to the Chairman of the Medical Manpower Committee at Addenbrooke's seeking permission to appoint an additional Consultant Cardiothoracic surgeon at Papworth with an interest in transplantation to start in July 1981. Half of this appointment was to be paid for by transplant funds and the other half would be a proleptic replacement for Christopher Parish who was due to retire in the spring of 1982. In the event, and after much wrangling, this was approved and John Wallwork joined us in November 1981, having gained valuable experience in the use of cyclosporine and heart-lung transplantation while Chief Resident at Stanford. John had previously been a locum senior registrar in Glasgow during which Philip Caves had spoken enthusiastically about him. I was keen to get help both with the increasing volume of coronary artery surgery and the heart transplant programme and after Philip's death I invited John to come and see me. He responded favourably and the result was that we appointed him to a senior registrar post for two months before he was due to spend a year with Dr Shumway, and it was towards the end of this period that he was appointed a consultant at Papworth.

While we were gaining valuable additions to our surgical staff, we lost our local cardiological support when, in September 1980, Michael Petch withdrew from further involvement in the heart transplant programme. This was a bitter blow, which I felt was mainly a result of the never-ending pressure he had been subjected to by his colleague David Evans. Michael also asked that his name be removed as co-author of our paper "Recent experience with heart transplantation", which was to be published in the British Medical Journal on 13th September and which was an account of the first 12 patients transplanted at Papworth. However, again I was to receive an unexpected and welcome letter of support from Professor John Goodwin, saying that he knew of many within the cardiological community who wanted to see the work at Papworth go ahead and that if I ever needed a second opinion with a difficult assessment he would be happy to provide this. So we continued at Papworth with surgeons and radiologists taking on the heart biopsies and many of the investigations previously done by cardiologists.

I was again invited to give an account of what had been happening at Papworth to the Transplant Advisory Panel meeting on 1st October. The favourable early results described in our article in the British Medical Journal paper had been circulated with the papers. Also on the agenda was an irritating letter from Peter Morris on behalf of the British Transplantation

Society to Sir Henry Yellowlees, the Chief Medical Officer, stating: "The British Transplantation Society is concerned that cardiac transplantation has recommenced in the UK without appropriate planning and funding by the DHSS", and concluding with "any unit considering the establishment of a programme should consult with the Transplant Advisory Panel before proceeding with planning". As if we had not been meticulous in doing just that!

Besides Dr Petch's withdrawal from the programme, another low point occurred towards the end of 1980 with a Panorama programme that had the pejorative title "Transplants: Are the donors really dead?" I suspect, though cannot be sure, that this was initiated by David Evans. In any event it proved to be the height of journalistic irresponsibility and, by casting doubt in the minds of the public as to the reliability of the diagnosis of brain-stem death, had a serious impact on all organ donations for at least the next six months.

However, our work continued and a year later in October 1981 the DHSS provided funds for a three-year research project to study the costs and benefits of the heart transplant programmes at Papworth and Harefield. This was under the direction of Martin Buxton from the Department of Health Economics at Brunel University and Professor Roy Acheson from the Department of Community Medicine in Cambridge, and its strength lay in its independence from the two clinical teams. Initially the Department had wanted a study of costs only, but prompted by us the researchers wisely insisted that benefits in terms of duration and quality of life after transplantation should also be included. I believe it was information concerning the latter that impressed both public and politicians when the final report was published at the end of 1984. The report also provided an impressive example of how new technologies should be evaluated before their more general introduction into the NHS, as evidenced by the following concluding statements:

"We are left with little doubt of the effectiveness of the procedure in terms of improvement in the quality and quantity of life of transplanted patients. But the value of these benefits must be compared with the value of the potential benefits to other perhaps quite different patients. The evidence of this report should help to make that comparison easier. It is not for us to prejudge in whose favour the comparison will be. But hopefully it will help to prevent demands for resources from services of un-assessed benefit and cost, depriving the transplant programmes of resources that they can clearly use to benefit their patients."

In due course, the report led to favourable consideration of the two transplant programmes at Papworth and Harefield and for secure and adequate funding under the Supra-Regional Services Scheme. This had been initiated by the DHSS in 1983 to first designate and then fund from central top-sliced monies those few specialist services which, in order to be economically viable and clinically effective, needed to be provided for populations substantially larger than any one Health Region. This was an excellent scheme, because once designation had been achieved we were able to include the occasional capital scheme for funding, and also calculate the next year's revenue budget on what we predicted could be achieved with our existing resources. In this way funding for heart-lung transplantation was made available after we started this in 1984. It also provided a mechanism for controlling the growth of new transplant centres in other parts of the country because any new programme had to be assessed, approved and designated before central funding was made available. Certainly as interest in heart transplantation developed rapidly from the mid 1980s onwards, I became aware of colleagues in other countries who envied the system of control we had in Britain as they saw far too many small programmes springing up in the most unlikely centres, whereas we concentrated our efforts in a small number of comparatively large units where best use could be made of scarce donors and other resources.

The expansion of the transplant programme at Papworth brought many benefits in its wake. Because of its rather isolated situation 12 miles west of Cambridge, there had always been intermittent difficulties with recruitment of nurses, particularly in the Intensive Care Unit. But as the hospital became better known this proved less of a problem. Similarly, we began to get excellent applicants for our surgical training posts. John Wallwork and I had similar views about the value of teaching operative technique under direct supervision. Coronary artery surgery was an ideal procedure for practising this and, if we were not personally doing the operation, we would always be present to assist the trainee and to ensure it was carried out correctly. They understood that if things were going too slowly, or becoming too difficult, we would simply swap sides and take over. I had never been exposed to anything like this during my own training, where the custom was either to assist the boss or be asked to get on with it on your own and let him know if you needed help. At Papworth I always found it fascinating to see how quickly new and relatively inexperienced trainees developed their skills. They might start off by being embarrassed at exposing their lack of technique, but having overcome this, and with the confidence of our presence as both teacher and support, they learned fast and within a matter of months had usually developed good technical skills. But good surgery requires good judgement as well as good technique and good judgement takes longer to acquire. The latter is based on both experience and character and this is where the "apprenticeship" component of surgical training comes in. Certainly I found the relationship between trainer and trainee to be one of the most rewarding aspects of my professional career and it has been a great pleasure in retirement to see how many of our Papworth trainees subsequently achieved leadership positions within the specialty of cardiac surgery.

However, to return to the Transplant programme. With John Wallwork and Richard Cory-Pearce there were now three of us to share the transplant work. I retained responsibility for assessing all patients referred for transplantation. Because of our lack of cardiology input I used to arrange for most of the invasive investigations to be carried out at the referring hospital so that patients only needed to be in Papworth for four or five days. They would then be returned to their own hospital, where they would wait until being called for transplantation or sent home if well enough. In either instance we required regular reports so that if there were a rapid deterioration we could give them more priority on the waiting list. In this aspect of the work I was greatly helped by our excellent social worker, Virginia O'Brien, whom I managed to fund from the transplant budget. The assessment procedure was that the patient would be admitted to the Surgical Unit and the accompanying spouse, relative or friend accommodated in one of two houses that we had bought in the village. Besides being used for this purpose, these houses were also available to relatives of patients who were recovering from transplantation, and sometimes by transplant patients who came from far afield and who we wanted to keep an eye on before sending home. So eventually a small transplant community became part of Papworth Village, rather like - although on a smaller scale – the relatives of patients being treated for tuberculosis by Sir Pendrill Varrier-Jones at Papworth in the 1920s and 1930s.

Soon after their admission I would see the patient in the presence of their accompanying spouse or relative. I would take a full medical history and review all the relevant investigations. I would also talk to them about the associated risks and benefits of heart transplantation, emphasising the unpredictability of the donor supply and the probability of episodes of rejection after a transplant, which might necessitate readmission to hospital during the first six to twelve months but which thereafter would become much less common. I also explained that they would always need to take drugs to suppress the immune system and that we would call them for follow up fairly regularly during the first year and thereafter at annual intervals when they would have a comprehensive review. This would include biopsy of the heart and an Xray study of the arteries in the transplanted heart, as we knew these could be affected by a process of narrowing in a proportion of survivors. The patients used to call this their "MOT". I also gave them in simple but accurate terms our up to date overall survival figures, illustrating that mortality was highest during the first year but that thereafter the situation improved with no more than a 5% chance of death per annum. I informed them about our Waiting List and how it operated. Patients were placed on it in chronological order but when a donor heart became available I allocated it after taking into consideration three other factors, namely blood group, size compatibility between donor and recipient, and urgency. In other words, if we knew of a patient who was deteriorating fast despite full medical treatment, we might transplant them ahead of someone who had been waiting longer.

This was a lot of information to impart during a single consultation, hence the importance of being accompanied by a relative and the availability afterwards of Virginia O'Brien to fill in gaps in their understanding. She would also introduce the patient to ward staff and other departments in the hospital with whom they would be likely to come in contact. They would also meet the transplant co-ordinators who had the important role of getting in touch with the patient when a donor heart became available for them. So before the days of mobile phones, they needed to be supplied with a "Pager" to be retained at all times if they were out of touch with their home telephone. At the end of the four or five days, I would have access to all the investigations performed during their admission and would see them for a final consultation. During this we would go over what they had learned during their stay concerning the implications of a transplant and all that this involved. If they remained keen to proceed and if I judged them to be sick enough and without any contra-indications, I would offer to place them on the waiting list. In some instances, if I felt someone had serious heart disease which was likely to progress but which at the time of assessment did not warrant transplantation, I placed them on a provisional list whereby they would be kept under observation by their own hospital and referred back to us for re-assessment if their condition deteriorated.

There was often considerable anxiety before this final consultation, accompanied by a great relief if they were accepted for transplantation. But then the difficult period of waiting for the transplant commenced. Most patients described this as stressful, even though they had been warned what to expect. If they were in their local hospital we would insist on regular reports of their condition. If at home, Virginia or one of the transplant co-ordinators would keep in touch to emphasise that they were not being forgotten. The patients also knew that I used to carry the waiting list around with me wherever I went, so that if I was informed that a donor heart was likely to become available I could arrange for an appropriate recipient to be brought to Papworth straight away. Sometimes this resulted in a false alarm, which was tough on the patient, but again we had explained why a speedy admission was necessary as the logistics of timing the donor operation to the recipient operation was not always easy. This was because once brain death had been confirmed the Intensive Care Unit in which the donor was being nursed usually wished the donor operation to be performed as expeditiously as possible. Also, coordination had to be achieved with surgical teams retrieving other organs such as the kidneys and liver. It varied from time to time but on average about one third of our patients died on the waiting list before a heart became available for them. I gave this statistic to them during their assessment as I knew it was something they would be concerned about and felt that they would prefer to know roughly what their chances were of being transplanted. It was striking how often I was informed by relatives of those patients who died without a transplant, that the extra hope they had received had made up for what was otherwise a hopeless situation.

When Richard Cory-Pearce was appointed he was given responsibility for running the Out Patients Clinic and arranging the necessary investigations for returning patients. In his role as British Heart Foundation Senior Research Fellow he therefore had the opportunity for collecting a lot of data and doing some interesting research projects. He did the work but unfortunately had difficulty in writing this up and publishing it. However, he was a good technical surgeon and soon able to do transplants on his own. I continued to do many of the donor operations during the first few years, knowing that a good early outcome depended on transplanting a good heart. John Wallwork was responsible for the post-operative management of patients whilst they were in hospital and he also did his share of transplants. At the same time our animal research continued at Huntingdon Research Centre, where John and I did a series of baboon heart-lung transplants in preparation for a clinical programme. During his stay at Stanford John had become familiar with heart-lung transplantation and had assisted Bruce Reitz at the first successful case. I therefore gave him responsibility for developing the programme at Papworth and on 5th April 1984 he did the first successful heart-lung transplant in Europe.

At the same time as these developments were taking place the demand for routine adult cardiothoracic surgery was increasing. Because we were a single specialty hospital we were able to adapt and plan for expansion in a focussed and efficient way. Additional operating rooms were commissioned and the Intensive Care Unit extended. Frank Wells, who had been our registrar, joined us as consultant in 1985 when Ben Milstein retired, and a few years later Sam Nashef and Steven Large were appointed. So I came to be surrounded by a very talented group of young surgeons all of whom had their special interest. However, we tried and I believe succeeded, in developing a strong team approach which was of great benefit, and not always evident in other units around the country. Anaesthetic staffing increased to keep up with the surgical workload and here again relations between colleagues remained excellent.

We were also for the most part blessed with good managers. The NHS had always been lightly managed with a much lower proportion of the health budget spent on management than in most countries. In the mid 1980s Margaret Thatcher decided it should be run in a more business-like way and commissioned the ex-head of Marks and Spencer to look into the matter. This resulted in the Griffiths Report and the introduction of "general management" into the health service. Many professionals found the new and energetic breed of managers difficult to deal with. Our policy, which generally worked, was to meet the newly appointed Chief Executive and make it clear that we regarded our responsibility was to give patients the best possible treatment whereas, amongst others, his was to provide us with the best working environment in which to achieve this.

As the transplant programme at Papworth became better known and as interest in heart transplantation gathered pace world wide, I began to receive requests from friends and colleagues in other countries to arrange training in transplantation for promising young surgeons who would then return and be responsible for establishing the procedure in their own department. This proved to be an additional source of excellent trainees. Sometimes we could offer them locum senior registrar posts, as with Phillip Spratt and Don Esmore from Australia, and Phillipe Despins and Jean-Paul Coutielle from France, each of whom spent a year with us. On other occasions they came as Fellows assigned to the transplant programme, during which they would usually also conduct some research. Then there were the more senior colleagues who came to see what we were doing, either before starting their own programme, in which case they often brought other members of their team with them, or just to see what we were up to and compare our procedures with theirs. Successful examples of the former were Chawalit Ongcharit from Bangkok who returned to perform the first successful heart transplant in South East Asia, and Zbigniew Religa who started a very active programme in Poland. Religa, who became a good friend, smoked more cigarettes a day than any man I have ever known. He went on to become well known in Poland and a few years before his death in 2008 he was urged to stand as an Independent for the Presidency of the country but without success.

Other visitors to Papworth during this time are too numerous to name individually. But four who gave me particular pleasure were Norman Shumway to whom I owed so much; John Kirklin my previous mentor from Birmingham, Alabama; Denton Cooley from Houston, Texas and Charles Cabrol from Paris.

I also did a lot of travelling, partly through invitations and partly to keep up with what others were doing. Interest in heart transplantation had grown rapidly after it was recognised that cyclosporine-based immunosuppression reduced both the frequency and intensity of early rejection episodes. As one who had been early in the field and with our very active programme at Papworth, I was invited to participate in many Overseas Visiting Professorships and Lectureships. Indeed I took part in no fewer than 31 of these between 1979 and 1989, during which time I also gave over a hundred lectures on transplantation and related subjects in the United Kingdom. One of the most interesting transplant meetings I attended during this time was in Rome in May 1989. Both Norman Shumway and Chris Barnard had been invited and they ended up being required to be joint chairmen for one of the sessions. Shumway looked uncomfortable throughout having steadfastly avoided meeting Barnard for

22 years since he had been pipped at the post by Barnard performing the world's first heart transplant on 3 December 1967. At the end of the session Shumway tried to escape as quickly as possible, but not before this historic photograph of the two men was taken, which was sent to me later by Chris Barnard. A happier Shumway is reflected in the adjoining photograph, taken with Magdi Yacoub, John Wallwork and me at the opening of the new Transplant Unit at Papworth in July 1998

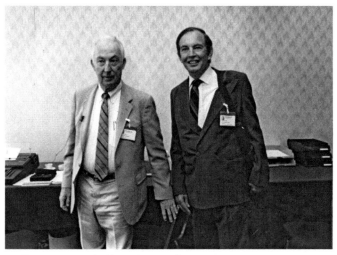

Norman Shumway and Chris Barnard at a meeting in Rome, May 1989.

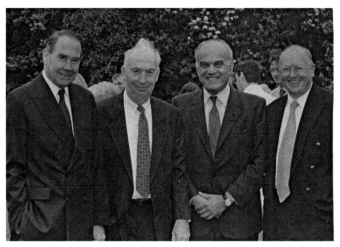

Norman Shumway and Magdi Yacoub with John Wallwork and me, July 1998. However, when I look back on the whole transplant experience, I can see that it is the early years from 1979 to the mid-1980's that were undoubtedly the most satisfying of my professional career. If I try and analyse why this should have been so I believe it is because they offered the opportunity to provide a complete package of care for the sick and anxious patients who were referred to us for transplantation. As in all medicine, it is the initial consultation between patient and doctor that can establish the trust and confidence that is so central to the whole endeavour. And how much more important this was for a group of patients who were being asked to accept a journey into the unknown. As mentioned, we told them all we could about the uncertainties of the donor supply, the risks and imponderables of the procedure itself and the possibility of rejection and infection. Although some of these concepts were complicated, it did seem possible with sympathy and a degree of optimism – to which surely all patients should be exposed – to achieve the sort of trust which meant so much not only to the patients but also to their wives, husbands or relatives. They also knew that if they were accepted for transplantation they would have our total commitment towards a successful outcome. Here again there was something about the Papworth environment that was so important. For they could see that everyone they came in contact with, from Virginia O'Brien to the Ward nursing staff, to the ECG technicians, the physiotherapists and even the ward auxiliaries, were interested in their survival and well being. I doubt this spirit could ever have been achieved in a large teaching hospital and curiously I think it was partly because for so much of the time our backs were against the wall as a result of inadequate and uncertain funding and criticism from the cardiologists and others that this increased the dedication and commitment to our patients. This spirit of determination, of not giving up, spilled over into the management of patients, each of whom was so precious to us and it was a summation of all these factors which visitors and teams from other parts of the world recognised as something special and which came to be called "The Papworth Experience".

I had been elected President of the Royal College of Surgeons in April 1989 and started my three year Presidency in July, at which time I passed on leadership of the transplant programme to John Wallwork. By then we had done 342 heart transplants and 68 heart-lung transplants. Of the former, one year survival had improved from 75% to 83% and ten year actuarial survival to 55%, with eleven of the first 100 patients living for more than twenty years. This was an excellent prospect for those who, without transplantation, could not have been expected to live more than six to twelve months at most. And although all patients had to remain permanently on drugs to suppress the immune system, and although these would sometimes give rise to nasty complications, the general quality of life amongst survivors was gratifyingly good. Many got back to work, some had babies, others had the pleasure of watching their children or grandchildren grow up. Papworth had given them the extra life that they valued and there was a strong bond between survivors and the hospital and staff who had looked after them. This was reflected during the celebrations which took place on 19th June 2004 when several hundred of the more than 1,000 heart transplants which had been performed by then returned to the hospital for the 25th Anniversary of the start of the programme. It was a huge pleasure to be there with them and to be presented with such striking evidence that all the hard work, difficulties and disappointments had in the end been worth it.

Chapter 6
The General Medical Council;
the Artificial Heart, and Private
Practice

Settling in Cambridge

On starting the locum post at Papworth in November 1972 I rented a small apartment in Cambridge. This was in Woodlark Road and to get there I had to drive through Sherlock and Eachard Roads. All three roads were named after Masters of St Catharine's College but of course at the time I was oblivious of the significance of this. With Ann and the four children still in London, it was agreed that I should be on-call on Monday, Tuesday, Wednesday and Thursday and that Ben would take care of the weekends, so that I could spend these with the family in Blackheath. When I was appointed to the substantive post in February 1973, we decided that the children should remain in London until the end of the school year, so this arrangement continued until the end of June when we all moved into rented accommodation in St Margaret's Road, Girton. Soon thereafter I found what I knew would be the perfect home for us. This was 19 Adams Road, a fine Edwardian building with a delightful garden, conveniently placed for schools and access to the centre of Cambridge. There were, however, two problems. Firstly the owner, Douglas Gairdner, who was the retiring senior paediatrician at Addenbrooke's, was unhappy about the idea of selling to a colleague, and secondly the lease of the property was owned by St John's College and only had 28 years to run. For this reason my solicitor was very much against the purchase, commenting that at the end of life a man's wealth resided largely in the property he owned. He thought me somewhat frivolous when I replied that I wanted the house and that with any luck I might expire at about the same time as the lease.

He also pointed out that it would be very unlikely I would ever be able to acquire the freehold. But in this he was wrong as the law changed five years later and we were able to purchase this from St John's. I also managed to win over Douglas Gairdner by being prepared to defer occupation until the alterations to his new house had been completed. This wasn't until a few weeks before Christmas but the wait was worth it and 19 Adams Road provided an extremely happy and convenient home for us for the next 20 years. Being on the west side of Cambridge I had an easy and pleasant journey to and from Papworth. Also Ann, who had been enjoying London whilst living in Blackheath, and who initially was not enthusiastic about the move, came to love Cambridge and made many new friends.

Developments at Papworth

Professional demands soon came to occupy a great deal of my time. It was clear to me that if Papworth were to survive as a Regional Cardiothoracic Unit the cardiac surgical activity would need to be substantially increased. Thoracic surgery was well served in Norwich by two surgeons, Findlay Kerr and Barry Ross and Ben Milstein and occasionally Chris Parish also did thoracic surgery at Papworth. But the open-heart programme, which they had started in the early '60s had never flourished and indeed in 1972 the activity was amongst the lowest in the country. One of the problems lay in the Intensive Care Unit where there were insufficient beds and nurses. We were soon able to expand the former and with various inducements nurse recruitment improved. There were two excellent anaesthetists, one of whom, Don Bethune, had a strong interest in developing the technology associated with the heart-lung machine, which supports the patient's circulation while the heart is being operated on. The cardiologists, Hugh Fleming and David Evans, were conservative and sometimes difficult and cardiac referrals improved when Ian Brooksby was appointed at Norwich. During the year 1974 we increased our open heart operations to 162 with an overall operative mortality of just under 5% and I took to sending a breakdown of our annual results to all physicians in the East Anglian Region to convince them that cardiac surgery could be accomplished with a high degree of safety.

At the beginning of 1975 I was approached by two cardiologists in Bristol who suggested I might be interested in a consultant post arising from the retirement of Ronald Belsey. On the face of it this seemed unattractive. I was enjoying my work at Papworth and as a family we had settled well into Cambridge. However, on further investigation it seemed that the

Bristol job offered tremendous potential. It served a much larger Region than East Anglia, the cardiologists were excellent and it included paediatric cardiac surgery, which I was keen to develop and which was largely absent at Papworth. I paid several visits to Bristol and soon came to realise that a serious deficiency was lack of sufficient operating space and time, and inadequate intensive care facilities. Having pointed this out I received various assurances that this would be dealt with. However, I remained sufficiently uncertain as to whether these would be provided, that a few days before the appointment I contacted the Professor of Surgery and asked for confirmation in writing that if appointed I would have access to five dedicated operating sessions per week. I went to Bristol the day before the interviews for further discussions but as I had received no written confirmation by noon the next day I returned to Cambridge. This was much to the relief of Ben Milstein and my dear wife, who did not look forward to another move.

Another similar proposal cropped up eighteen months later when I was asked by John Dark to consider an appointment in Manchester to help expand the work at Wythenshawe Hospital. However, by then Ann and I had become so impressed with the social advantages of living in Cambridge and I had become sufficiently committed to developing the heart transplant programme that it was not difficult to say No.

The UK Cardiac Surgical Register
To keep up to date I continued my practice of visiting colleagues in other centres to see them at work and learn from them. I also enjoyed assisting Donald Ross with his private patients in London when I had a Saturday morning free. He was at the height of his powers and besides being a fine clinician was one of the best technical surgeons I ever worked with. These visits led me to take an interest in what was going on in cardiac surgery in the rest of the country. I had recently come across a report from the Australian Heart Foundation in which the type and number of all heart operations were recorded each year, together with the in-hospital mortality for each category and decided that something similar would be of benefit to the United Kingdom. So I obtained permission from the Executive Council of the Society of Cardiothoracic Surgeons of Great Britain and Ireland, to which I had just been elected, to undertake what I described as a 'pilot' study. What I hadn't made clear was that I intended to seek information from all of the 44 Units then practising cardiac surgery in the UK. I made some slight modifications to the forms being used for the

Australian register and then sent these with a request to either the senior surgeon or one who I knew to fill in the data for their Unit and then return this to me At this stage I felt it would be better to ask for the cumulative results from each Unit rather than surgeon specific data. I was pleased to receive completed returns from 76% of those distributed and there was great interest when the results were presented at the next annual meeting of the Society. Besides illustrating how many of each type of cardiac operation was being performed in the country, surgeons could compare their own mortality figures for specific operations with the national average. I was also able to present "scattergrams" showing how hospital mortality for common operations varied between different units and the relationship of this to throughput. Apart from other considerations, such information had powerful educational implications, for if your Unit had a substantially higher operative mortality for a particular operation, there would be a strong incentive to find out why and then try and correct this. As a result of what was shown, the Society agreed that an annual UK Cardiac Surgical Register should be established to which every Unit would be required to contribute. I was asked to help with this and the Secretary of the Society, John Dark, and I were given overall responsibility for data collection and analysis and the publication of an Annual Report. This was to contain national data on the number of operations performed and the average hospitality mortality for each category. We secured the help of Dr Alan Bailey at BUPA for statistical analysis and every Unit received a copy of the Report after the end of each year. We had some trouble to start with as a result of a small number of Units being late with submitting their data, thereby holding up analysis, and one year there were two who failed to contribute. However, this was corrected by a resolution passed at the next annual meeting whereby any Unit failing to submit their data would be named in that year's Report. The Register continued to persist in its original form for a decade until the mid-1980s, after which the Society embarked upon a more sophisticated analysis of activity with risk-adjusted mortality data. More recently, and not without a degree of controversy, members of the Society agreed to the public release of surgeon-specific results. In this way, I believe our specialty has led the way with respect to transparency over the performance and quality outcomes of its membership.

Election to the Council of the Royal College of Surgeons

As a result of my involvement with the UK Cardiac Surgical Register I became relatively well known within the specialty of cardiothoracic surgery. Further attention came my way from surgeons in other specialties because of the heart transplant programme. However, it still came as a surprise when at the beginning of 1981 I was asked by the then President of the Society of Cardiothoracic Surgeons, Jack Belcher, if I would be prepared to be nominated for election to the Council of the Royal College of Surgeons of England. Being still relatively junior I agreed to this in the belief that it would be highly unlikely as council members were elected by the whole Fellowship of the College, numbering more than 5,000 surgeons. Interestingly, I bumped into Donald Ross soon after this and he mentioned he was considering standing for Council. When I told him what had happened he immediately threw his application form into the waste paper basket, saying he wouldn't want to split the cardiac surgical vote and he was not too keen anyway. What a response from one of my most revered mentors! I took no further interest in events until on the afternoon of the election I received a telephone call from the President's secretary. This occurred while I was in a rather seedy television studio in Soho, where I was reviewing the 'rushes' of a film about the transplant programme at Papworth. I had agreed to this being made because the Central Office for Information had been commissioned by the Foreign Office for the film to be distributed abroad, confirming it would not be shown in the UK. When the President of the College, Sir Alan Parks, was put through he congratulated me and much to my surprise said that I had been elected by a substantial majority. This was in April and he suggested I make an appointment to see him but that I would not be required to attend my first Council meeting until July, which was the start of the college year. The election was for eight years with permission to stand for an extra four providing one was within the age limit. Thus began my long and valued association with the Royal College of Surgeons.

At that time Council comprised twenty-four members elected by the whole Fellowship of the College from whom the President and two Vice-Presidents were elected by secret ballot. The President served for three years and the Vice-Presidents for two. In addition the Deans of the Faculties of Anaesthetists and Dental Surgery served on Council and there were representatives from the Royal Colleges of Obstetricians and Gynaecologists, Radiologists, and General Practitioners. The Secretary of the College, Ronald Johnson-Gilbert, was an immensely impressive person and amongst his many other duties was responsible for the agenda and minutes of all major meetings. Council in Committee met in the morning, when reports were received and discussed from the various college committees. The more formal meeting of Council took place in the afternoon, during which gowns were worn and members stood to speak and were only permitted to speak once on any particular agenda item. The President or chairman of the committee presenting the report would then sum up and if it was perceived there was a sufficient consensus the motion was agreed and passed. Very rarely was a vote resorted to. A Council Club dinner was held in the evening at quarterly intervals. This had been founded in 1869 and the dinner I attended after my first Council meeting was the 407th meeting of the Club. Only past and present members of Council attended and the format was for a new member of Council to be in the chair for the evening. Towards the end of the meal the Secretary would read the minutes of the last meeting and then someone would give an introductory speech about the chairman, who would then rise and talk about himself for about twenty minutes, after which a toast was drunk. The custom was to be fairly revealing about oneself and not concentrate just on achievements. I was fascinated by the first dinner I attended, which was held in the splendid oak-lined Council room with the college silver on display. I thought the chairman's speech was interesting but at the end of it the elderly orthopaedic surgeon who had been sitting next to me said in a loud hoarse whisper "too bloody long" and walked out. This was an important reminder not to exceed twenty minutes when I took the Chair the following year.

Alan Parks was very good to me. He recognised that I was extremely busy at Papworth and said that initially I would be spared a heavy committee burden but I should always attend Council meetings. This I was happy to do. I was also fortunate in that he invited me to join him at the quarterly Joint Meetings of the Surgical Colleges. These were held on a rotating basis at each of the four Royal Surgical Colleges in England, Edinburgh, Glasgow and Ireland and were attended by the President and two representatives from each college. The purpose of the meetings was to discuss issues needing collaboration between the colleges of which the two main ones at that time were examinations and the role of the surgical specialty associations. Each college had its own Fellowship examination and these needed to be comparable. However, there was a strong feeling amongst our Court of Examiners that the Irish and two Scottish colleges had made theirs easier in order to attract candidates and hence income from the lifelong subscriptions of those who passed. As mentioned, during my training I had taken both the English and the Edinburgh FRCS exams. Having been failed I thought somewhat unfairly in the former, I had gone straight to Edinburgh where I was certainly treated more professionally and where the clinical part of the examination seemed superior to what I had experienced in London. I did, however, still want to have the English FRCS and so took it again on the next occasion and passed. The issue with the surgical specialty associations was that the FRCS of one of the four colleges was required for entry into higher surgical training. Thereafter, however, the tendency was for surgeons to become more involved with the society representing their specialty than with the college in which they held their Fellowship. It had always seemed to me illogical for someone not to be examined in the specialty he or she was to be engaged in for the rest of their professional life and Edinburgh had begun to look at the prospect of holding such examinations. I was a strong supporter of this but felt that as the specialty associations drew their membership from across the United Kingdom and Ireland such examinations should be intercollegiate in nature, with examiners coming from all four colleges. The specialty associations were growing in power and influence and were themselves adamant that if such examinations were to be held towards the end of training there should only be one for each specialty rather than each college having one of their own. We were further ahead than the other colleges in wanting to embrace the surgical specialties, which we finally achieved in 1989 by agreeing to have the President of each of the nine specialty associations as an invited member of Council, where they were able to participate fully in Council affairs, except for voting for the President and Vice-Presidents. As might be imagined conduct of these Joint Meetings of Surgical Colleges did not always run smoothly. Alan Parks was greatly respected by the other presidents and for me it was an invaluable experience both in surgical politics and in getting to know senior members of the other three colleges. Sadly, Alan's tenure as President was cut short when he had a serious heart attack whilst at a meeting in Rome in October 1982. I flew out to assess the situation and to be with his wife Caroline. He was being nursed in an Intensive Care Unit and was keen to return to England as soon as possible. However, at the time he was too unstable to move and it was not until a week later on 3rd November that I was able to bring him back to England in a Lear Jet paid for by the College I was accompanied by my anaesthetist from Papworth, Don Bethune, and the senior registrar in cardiology from Bart's where Alan wished to be taken. Caroline accompanied us in the plane and I was relieved when we were able to deliver him safely into the hands of Roworth Spurrell, the senior cardiologist at St Bartholomew's Hospital. He underwent immediate coronary angiography followed by a coronary bypass graft operation by my friend, Gareth Rees, the same evening. Sadly, however, he had very extensive disease and never recovered from the operation, a great loss to British surgery as well as to the College. Geoffrey Slaney was elected his successor, with whom I again developed excellent relations. Inevitably as the decade progressed and I became more senior on Council the demands from the College increased so that by 1988 I was chairing the Board of Surgical Training and the Fellowship Election and Prize Committee, as well as being a member of the Executive Committee, the Finance and General Purposes Committee and the Fund-Raising Committee. There were also some social occasions I was required to attend and all this had to be accommodated within increasing demands from Papworth and a busy private practice at the Wellington Hospital in London of which more anon.

The General Medical Council

Another interesting and educational experience was service on the General Medical Council (GMC) from 1983 to 1989. This, I believe, was the result of Ronald Johnson-Gilbert's advocacy, as I remember a conversation with him after I had been on Council about two years. He said he thought it would provide insight into a broad spectrum of issues affecting the medical profession and that perhaps I ought to be the College's representative on the GMC, which duly came about. At that time Council had a membership of about 110 and met formally twice a year under the Presidency of Sir John (later Lord) Walton. Much of the work of the GMC was done by the main committees between Council meetings. These included the Registration Committee which was responsible for holding the list of Registered Medical Practitioners; the Education Committee which had statutory responsibility for overseeing all medical education, including inspecting those medical schools whose graduates could be registered with the GMC; the Standards Committee, and the two disciplinary committees, the Preliminary Proceedings Committee and the Professional Conduct Committee. My first commitment was to the former, whose role was to receive and review all complaints made to the GMC by members of the public or medical profession. Having received a complaint there were four options open to the committee. These were either to dismiss it; to send 'a letter of admonition' to the doctor complained against; to refer the doctor to the Health Committee if there seemed to be a psychiatric problem or drug or alcohol abuse; or finally to refer the individual to the Conduct Committee where he or she would undergo a formal trial at the end of which the judgement would be either guilty or not guilty of "serious professional misconduct". If the former the doctor would be struck off the medical register or have restrictions applied to his or her registration. The problem with this system was that there was no disciplinary category between a 'letter of admonition' and 'serious professional misconduct'. Hence there was no way of disciplining doctors who might be guilty of quite serious incompetence but short of serious professional misconduct, which was left to the Courts. This issue was addressed as part of the radical reforms of the GMC that took place following Dame Janet Smith's report after the trial of Dr Shipman, who had been found guilty of murdering a large number of elderly patients over a long period of time without being detected.

My first meeting of the Preliminary Proceedings Committee (PPC) was a memorable one. During the preceding week I had received two large packets containing the files of the cases to be considered. I had waded through most of these by late Sunday evening and fortunately decided to travel to the meeting next morning by train, rather than by car, so that I could read the remaining few cases. One of these related to a young orthopaedic surgeon who had behaved badly at a hospital party, resulting in a complaint to the GMC by one of the nurses involved. After I had been welcomed by the chairman as a new member of the committee, he decided to take this case first and immediately asked my views on it. I can still recall the sense of relief that I had made time to read all the papers, as otherwise my credibility with the committee would have been seriously damaged at this my first meeting. In the event, my judgement was that he had been very foolish but that his behaviour did not warrant referral to the Conduct Committee. I was then dismayed when the only other surgeon on the committee, a very senior man, took precisely the opposite view. However, after further discussion, the majority opinion coincided with mine and he was sent a letter of admonition. As time went by I was thankful to be serving on the Preliminary Proceedings Committee rather than on the Professional Conduct Committee. The latter dealt with a relatively small number of cases, some of which might go on for several weeks, whereas the PPC received a large number of unfiltered complaints, some of which were serious and some not.

The composition of the GMC at that time, unlike now, had a heavy preponderance of medical members. There were some like me who represented colleges and other medical institutions, and there were a small number of appointed lay members, some of whom were very vociferous. The majority, however, were doctors elected on a regional basis covering the whole of the United Kingdom. Some of these had been 'sponsored' during their election by various organisations such as the British Medical Association and these tended to be the most political. The majority, however, stood as independent candidates and consequently embraced a wide range of opinion. John Walton was a superb President. Despite his other demanding commitments as Warden of Green College, Oxford, he was always well briefed and was highly respected by most members of Council for the wisdom and authority with which he presided over the debates.

Towards the end of my time on the GMC I served on the Education Committee, which again proved to be a fascinating experience. One of the topical issues was whether a change should be made to the Medical Register by including specialist certification. I spoke strongly in favour of this, which was consistent with our move towards introducing an exam at the end of specialist training. However, it was nearly a decade before this was finally achieved. In retrospect I found my six years on the Council to be most valuable. It exposed me to aspects of the medical profession that I had no previous experience of and it enabled me to make contacts and friends across a wide range of disciplines other than surgery, thereby widening my professional horizon.

The International Society for Heart Transplantation

Another institution I became involved with during the 1980s was the International Society for Heart Transplantation, of which I was a founder member. During my periodic visits to Stanford whilst preparing for the transplant programme in Cambridge I had become good friends with Stuart Jamieson. He was from Rhodesia initially and had trained at St Mary's Hospital and the Brompton Hospital in London before being awarded a British-American scholarship to do research at Stanford. When we first met he was working in Dr Shumway's laboratory testing various immunosuppressive regimes in rats, which seemed to me not the easiest animals to do heart transplants on. He later progressed to Chief Resident and then staff member on Shumway's Unit at Stanford. When in Palo Alto I used to stay with Stuart and his lovely Californian girlfriend, Libby, who he later married. We subsequently became lifelong friends and I am proud to be godfather to their daughter, Alexandra. He used to work incredibly hard and would be gone in the morning long before I rose at a more civilised hour. Their apartment in Menlo Park was a short distance from the University, and I loved my walk there through the beautiful oak-lined avenue. Everyone else seemed to be running, cycling or travelling by motorbike or car and seldom did I see another walker.

In October 1980 I received a letter from Stuart saying there was talk of an informal transplant group gathering at the American Heart Association meeting in Miami on 17th November to discuss cardiac transplantation and related issues. This was being organised by Michael Hess, who was Professor of Medicine at the Medical College of Virginia (MCV). Michael had attached a list of 15 individuals whom he knew to be currently active in cardiac transplantation and expressed his interest in forming a small group who would share protocols and gather data related to heart transplantation. He went on to write: "Personally I disagree with Dr Leaf's opinion, as editor of the New England Journal of Medicine, that no new scientific information is likely to emerge from the field of cardiac transplantation" and added that it was his opinion that the challenge of refuting this was "best met by slow, careful investigation and, because of the nature of involvement in cardiac transplantation, cooperative efforts between physicians and surgeons will be necessary". He also pointed out that Dr Andrea Hastillo at MCV had kindly agreed to serve as co-ordinating secretary and that if the meeting was successful we should perhaps regroup at the American College of Cardiology meeting in San Francisco in March 1981. Thus was born the concept of a society that, during the next decade and beyond, became of considerable importance to those teams developing heart transplant programmes around the world.

I was not able to be at the Florida meeting that was attended by seventeen representatives from Stanford, MCV, Mayo Clinic, Michael Reese Hospital Chicago, University of Minnesota, Arizona Health Sciences, University of Pittsburgh, Notre Dame Hospital Montreal and the National Hospital of Norway in Oslo. An inventory of transplant activity from eight institutions as of the date of that meeting yielded a total of 314 cases with 126 living. The majority came from Stanford (199 cases, 75 living), Cape Town (45 cases, 15 living), and MCV (39 cases, 12 living). By this time we had done 14 cases of which 8 were living. The pros and cons of shared protocols were discussed as was the need for a central registry for gathering meaningful data. A committee was established to determine what information should be included and this would be considered at the first meeting of what

Michael Hess now termed the "International Study Group for Cardiac Transplantation". This duly went ahead in San Francisco on 14th March 1981 with representatives from Montreal, Papworth, Paris and Munich in addition to those from the United States, thereby establishing the society's international character right from the beginning. An interesting scientific programme preceded a business meeting at which it was agreed that charter membership of what was now to be called the International Society for Heart Transplantation should be granted to those participants representing the eleven active programmes who had attended the meeting. Norman Shumway was elected Honorary Life President and Michael Hess President supported by a Secretary/Treasurer, Andrea Hastillo, and a small Executive Council. One of these was Jacques Losman, who was given the task of editing the proceedings of the meeting and he subsequently wrote to me asking for a contribution to the first number of the Proceedings of the Society with which I complied. He also mentioned that it was his intention to issue three or four numbers of the Proceedings each year. This proposal was regarded as being too ambitious by other members of the Executive Council but Jacques persisted in his objective and within a few months an Editorial Board had been formed of which I became a member. A contract was then signed on behalf of the Society with Professional Medical Services who agreed to publish a quarterly journal called "Heart Transplantation." This would be produced at their expense and they would be allowed to sell advertising space limited to ten pages per issue. Editorial control would remain with the Society and the Journal would be sent free to members of the Society and to a long list of other cardiologists and cardiac surgeons in the United States.

The second meeting took place in Phoenix, Arizona in May 1982. Jack Copeland, who had been at Stanford but was now in Phoenix, took over as President from Michael Hess and I was elected President-elect. The Society began to grow very rapidly and by the time of the third meeting, which was held in New Orleans in March 1983, we had presentations from many of the most active and influential individuals in the field of heart transplantation and cardiac assist devices. So by the time I took over as President at the end of the New York meeting in May 1984 the Society was well established. In keeping with its early, somewhat grandiose title, it had become truly 'International' and I was proud to be the first non-American President. A pleasing feature from the beginning had been its collegiality and multi-disciplinary nature. Surgeons, cardiologists, immunologists, pathologists, virologists and microbiologists, all had their contribution to make as, importantly, did nurses, transplant co-ordinators and technicians. With the advent of cyclosporine, and having learned how to use this in conjunction with other immunosuppressive agents, results improved and this sparked renewed interest in the potential of heart transplantation with a rapid increase in activity all over the world. During these early years I believe the Society provided an important role for communicating scientific advances and good practice, both through the publication of the Journal and the quality of the annual meetings. There was much to be excited about and many lasting friendships were made which enriched the years that followed. The only sad exception in this respect was my friendship with Jacques Losman. His relationship with the manager of Professional Medical Services had never been good and deteriorated to the extent that new publishers had to be found by the time our contract with them expired at the end of two years in September 1985. Jacques and his assistant, Dawn Griffiths, had effectively been running the Society but his Editorship of the Journal began to receive serious complaints. This was not entirely his fault as he never received the support from his Editorial Board that was his due and there is no doubt that he deserved great credit for having kept the Journal going under difficult circumstances. However, at the second New York meeting in 1986 it was decided by the Executive that Michael Kaye should take over as Editor and the respected firm of CV Mosby became the publishers. This inevitably came as a great disappointment to Jacques and was something over which he felt I should have supported him more strongly. For me it was a matter of considerable regret that my presidency, which had otherwise been hugely enjoyable, should have ended on this unhappy note. However, the Journal went from strength to strength. It soon became a monthly publication under its new title of 'The Journal of Heart and Lung Transplantation" and by the end of the long and distinguished editorship of Jim Kirklin, who had succeeded his father as Professor and Head of Cardiothoracic Surgery at the University of Alabama at Birmingham, it had become one of the most respected medical journals with a circulation of over three thousand. Stuart Jamieson succeeded me as President after the meeting in New York and was responsible for putting the affairs of the Society under professional management. By the time of the Thirtieth Anniversary in Chicago in April 2010, which I was unfortunately unable to attend (because of Icelandic volcanic dust preventing air travel) membership of the Society had grown to 2,400 of whom about 1,400 were present at the meeting.

The Artificial Heart

Another transplant related activity that I became involved with during the 1980s was experience with the Jarvik Artificial Heart. This had been designed in Willem Kolff's laboratories in Salt Lake City, Utah. Kolff had gained his reputation by constructing the world's first artificial kidney while in Holland during the Second World War. After the War he was attracted to the Cleveland Clinic in America where he began work on an artificial heart. It had long been recognised that however successful heart transplantation became, there would always be a mismatch between patients waiting for a heart and the availability of appropriate donor organs. It soon became clear that the only alternatives would lie in the use of either mechanical hearts or animal hearts. Problems with the latter, besides ethical considerations, resided in the strong way in which tissue is rejected when transplanted across species. The only solution to this seemed to be genetic modification of the animal in a way that would render its organs less likely to be rejected when transplanted into a human. And although progress has been made, this still remains a distant and difficult goal.

The concept of being able to take an appropriately sized artificial heart off the shelf and place it in a patient when needed, rather than having to wait for a donor heart to become available, is an attractive one. Two early problems were recognised in the design of artificial hearts. First there has to be biocompatibility between the patient's blood and the surfaces lining the interior of the heart, otherwise clots will form which might then be distributed to the brain and other vital organs. Then there is the problem of the power source to drive the heart. Here the options were compressed air, electricity, or nuclear. The first was the simplest but involves connecting the artificial heart via tubes exiting the body to a compressor and console alongside the patient, which would control the rate and output of the heart. If electricity were to be used as a power source this would necessitate connecting the heart via wires to an external power supply, but would have the potential advantage of intermittent connection to a portable battery worn in a harness on the body so that the patient could be more mobile. The ideal of course would be a totally implantable power source, leaving the patient free from all external connections. Here nuclear power seemed the only option but this was, and remains, too controversial for practical application.

I was aware of some of these developments and indeed can remember reading an article published by William Kolff in 1963 entitled "Today the

Calf; Tomorrow Man", in which he described his early experience with the artificial heart while at the Cleveland Clinic. However, it wasn't until 19 years later, on 1st December 1982, that Bill DeVries inserted a Jarvik artificial heart into the 64-year old dentist, Barney Clark, in Salt Lake City as a permanent implant. Robert Jarvik had been working with Kolff since the latter's move to Utah and the device used, which was pneumatically driven, owed much to Kolff's earlier design. Anyway, amidst great publicity, Barney Clark survived 112 days, during which time he suffered a number of strokes from blood clots arising from within the heart. However, it was clear that the artificial heart was able to provide an effective circulation and reverse the signs and symptoms of heart failure.

Like others involved in transplantation I took an interest in the course of these events but it came as a surprise when some months later I was phoned by Robert Jarvik, whom I had never met, to say that he was in London and would like to meet me. We arranged to have dinner at a restaurant near the Wellington Hospital in St John's Wood, during which he produced an artificial heart from one of his pockets. He then explained how effective it was and how its lining had been improved since the model used on Barney Clark and suggested that I might find an application for it in my transplant programme at Papworth. I responded by saying that I could only see it being used in a desperate situation with a patient near to death and no donor heart available, when it might be used as a temporary implant until a human heart became available. This reflected the fact that at the time about a third of our patients listed for transplantation died before a heart became available. Hence if it were to be used, I would confine its role to that of a "bridge-to-transplant" rather than as a permanent implant, as had been the case with Barney Clark. I also went on to observe that I doubted very much that I would ever be able to get the significant research funding needed for such a project. Jarvik pointed out that he had already considered this and that he believed the Humana Corporation might be a potential source of funding. By this time Bill DeVries had been tempted by Humana to leave his university post in Utah and join their large private hospital in Louisville, Kentucky. There, in conjunction with Alan Lansing, he had done two more artificial heart implants and although they had not been successful his activity had brought much good publicity to the hospital. Humana was predominantly based in America where it owned some ninety hospitals, but it had recently purchased the Wellington Hospital in London where, as I shall relate, I had become Director of Cardiac Surgery. Jarvik's intention seemed to be that Humana might fund a number of private cases if these were done in the Wellington. However, I was adamant that if I became involved it could only be within the NHS and that meant Papworth Hospital. After further discussions we agreed that I would go to Louisville to meet the two men who had started Humana and were then the majority shareholders. These were two relatively young law graduates from Louisville, Wendell Cherry and David Jones, of whom I had already heard good reports. On arrival in Louisville I was met by Bill DeVries who was most helpful and after demonstrating the artificial heart and the way it was operated, he explained some of the technical features associated with its implantation. He then stressed that if I were to go ahead with the project I would first need to train in its use by doing a series of animal operations in the laboratories in Utah. If the heart were to be used as a bridge-to-transplant, this would involve doing an implant in a calf and then returning about a month later to remove the artificial heart and replace it with a calf heart of appropriate size, during the whole of which time I would need the assistance of the local laboratory technicians. Clearly this was going to be a major undertaking so when I met Wendell Cherry and David Jones I explained this and said I thought I would need US$0.5 million to cover travel and training expenses for me and two colleagues plus costs related to equipment and hospital stay at Papworth for two or three cases. In return, all I could offer was appropriate publicity by acknowledging Humana's generosity towards the British National Health Service. This surprisingly they agreed to and everything was signed and sealed before my return to the UK a few days later. Such is the way that American private enterprise operates! I did, however, take the precaution of informing them that I would need to get ethical approval from the local health authority before proceeding.

So after return to Papworth and getting the support of my colleagues I made arrangements with Willem Kolff to start work at his laboratories. He seemed enthusiastic to see a new clinical application for the artificial heart and during the ensuing few months I made three visits to Salt Lake. One of these was with Don Esmore, who had been our senior registrar for a year and was soon to return to Sydney, and two were with my recently appointed colleague, Frank Wells, who I thought might play a major role in the artificial heart work when it came to Papworth. We were met with great kindness by Dr Kolff and he spent time instructing us in the history and problems he had encountered whilst developing the artificial heart. We saw less of Robert Jarvik, who was not always in town, and I gathered that relations between them were somewhat strained. The animal laboratories were extremely well equipped and staffed, and with the help of the knowledgeable technicians we were able to achieve survival after implantation of the heart in calves but never to complete successfully the more difficult second part of the experiment, in which the artificial heart was removed and replaced by a donor heart from another animal. However, after three visits I felt we had learned enough to use the device as a bridge-to-transplant in a human.

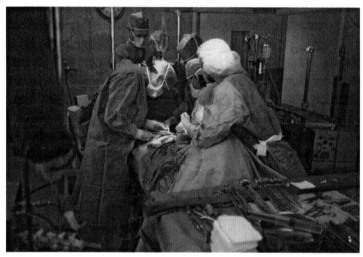

Inserting an artificial heart into a calf (Salt Lake City).

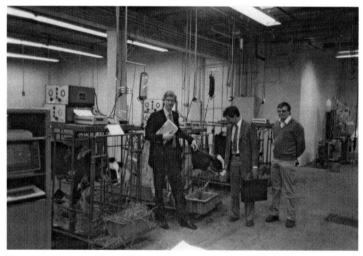

Calf the next day with artificial heart - Frank Wells, Don Esmore and Dereck Wheeldon looking on.

An important event occurred the day before departure of our final visit. Frank Wells and I had dinner with my very good friend from Canadian days, Frank Joklik, and his wife Pam. Frank was now based in Salt Lake City as President of Kennecott Copper Company, which amongst others owned the biggest open-cast copper mine in the world nearby. He was a keen skier and during the evening, and after much wine, suggested that we should all go skiing on Snowbird Mountain the next day. Frank Wells had never skied and my total experience was two weeks at Meribel in the French Alps twenty-five years earlier. However, the challenge was on and the next day we spent a glorious morning skiing Snowbird. Frank frightened Frank Joklik by spending much of the time going very fast straight downhill out of control, and I found that, rather as with riding a bicycle, what I had learned all those years earlier soon came back. Indeed my enjoyment was such that I determined from then on I would take my family skiing once a year. This is what we did and these holidays, usually accompanied by one or more of the children's friends, became very special to all of us. Just one of the many things I have Frank Joklik to be thankful for

Having gained the necessary ethical approval we trained our technicians at Papworth, Dereck Wheeldon and Roy Gill, how to drive the console but we then had a long wait before being referred a suitable patient. One of the main reasons for the delay was that the early model of the Jarvik heart was rather bulky and rigid and in previous cases there had been problems with closing the chest after the heart had been inserted. I therefore decided that our first patient needed to be of large size with a capacious chest. Eventually on 4th November 1986 one such patient was referred to me, having had a massive heart attack about ten days earlier. He was in low output heart failure and despite all pharmacological support was deteriorating fast, but still sufficiently conscious to be able to consent to the operation, with which his wife agreed. So we went ahead as soon as the necessary preliminary procedures had been completed, with Frank Wells and John Wallwork assisting me. Once the patient had been placed on the heart-lung machine, I excised the heart, leaving the posterior walls of the two collecting chambers, onto which we sewed two prosthetic atrial cuffs. These then had to be connected to the two plastic pumping chambers, supposedly by a 'quick-fit' mechanism, but which proved the most difficult part of the operation. The outlet tubes from the two pumps were then sewn respectively to the aorta and pulmonary artery. Finally the compressed air drive- lines, one for each of the pumps, were tunnelled through the rib cage and connected to the drive console. Having completed all the connections it was a great relief to see that the 'fit' was satisfactory and that the chest could be closed without difficulty. We now began to activate the pumps as we slowly reduced the flow from the heart-lung machine. We were able to adjust the volume of blood ejected with each beat by adjusting the pressure and flow of the compressed air activating the pumps, and also the rate at which the heart beat. It was a fascinating experience to have such total mechanical control over the amount of blood being pumped around the body and the patient was soon disconnected from the heart-lung machine. Having stopped any bleeding the chest was closed and the patient returned to the Intensive Care Unit where besides the regular nursing care our two technicians took it in turn to look after and adjust the operation of the drive console.

Altogether the whole procedure had gone more smoothly than I could have anticipated. The patient woke up within a few hours and was soon breathing on his own with evidence of a good cardiac output. Our Regional Press Officer John Edwards put out a Press statement, giving due recognition to Humana for their role in funding the whole endeavour. During the next two days I remained impressed with the performance of the artificial heart and was looking forward to stabilising the patient on it for at least a week or two, when I had a telephone call from my previous senior registrar, Chris McGregor, who was now head of the transplant unit in Newcastle. He told me he had been offered a donor heart that he felt sure would be suitable for my patient if it were the right blood group. This indeed was the case and I then had the difficult task of deciding whether to use it or not. On the one hand, suitable donor hearts of the right size and blood group were not going to be frequently available. On the other hand I would have preferred a longer period of stabilisation with the artificial heart before subjecting my patient to another major operation so soon after its insertion. In the event, it was not too difficult to decide that it was in the best interests of the patient to take the opportunity of exchanging the artificial heart for a human one, even though this had become available so much earlier than I would have wished. So I explained the situation to the patient and his wife and then after co-ordinating with Newcastle regarding the time of arrival of the donor heart at Papworth, back we went to the operating theatre. We started in early evening and it was a difficult procedure so that we didn't finish until about 3 am. However, there were no complications apart from some prolonged bleeding at the end of the operation and I drove home elated but very tired, only to be caught for speeding by an unsympathetic traffic policeman just as I entered Cambridge! Our patient had a more difficult recovery after his second operation but after leaving hospital he improved steadily and thereafter remained in good health until he died suddenly from an infection nearly two years later. And there ended the saga of my involvement with the Jarvik artificial heart. We had certainly shown that it could provide a satisfactory alternative circulation to the human heart. But it seemed to me that the procedures associated with using it as a bridge-to-transplant were just too complicated to be practical, as well as being very expensive, and that the future lay in developing mechanical devices which could be used to assist the failing heart without replacing it and left in-situ until a donor heart became available. This in fact is what has happened and there are now many devices on the market that fulfil this function. Some patients have been supported on them for many months and a few for more than two years. As far as the total artificial heart is concerned, the biocompatibility of the lining surfaces has been largely, though not completely solved, but a satisfactory wholly implantable power source has yet to be achieved. However, there still remain optimists in this difficult field, one such being Alain Carpentier in Paris, who recently presented details of a very sophisticated artificial heart that is nearing clinical trials. Jarvik himself gave up work on total artificial hearts after his device was banned for use in America, but then turned his talents towards making a very small assist device that has now been used widely. The original Jarvik heart which I inserted, together with the large drive console and related equipment now resides in the National Museum of Science and Industry in London to which it was donated when I retired from Papworth.

Lunch with the Queen

One of the most delightful and unexpected social events that occurred around this time (10th December 1986) was a personal invitation to have lunch with Her Majesty the Queen. On arrival at Buckingham Palace I found that I was one of eight guests. We were invited into a reception room where, after a short while, we were joined by the Queen accompanied by her two Corgis, and Princess Alexandra, who I thought was perhaps the most gracious and beautiful woman I had ever met. After drinks we proceeded to a small dining room where to my great surprise I found I was seated next to the Queen. We had been told beforehand that when addressing her for the first time one should use the term "Your Majesty", but that thereafter "Ma'am" was sufficient, and that normally it should be left to her to open a new subject of conversation.

After enquiring about my work at Papworth, about which she must have been informed, conversation lagged somewhat and so I rather hesitantly took it upon myself to reopen the conversation by saying: "You know, Ma'am, the first time I saw you was when I was a 15 year old schoolboy taking part in a gym display in Pietermaritzburg in your honour when you and your parents and Princess Margaret visited South Africa in 1947." This resulted in an animated account about what a wonderful experience that visit had been, how well they had been looked after by General Smuts, and what a joy it had been to have fresh fruit and an inexhaustible supply of chocolates after the privations of the war years in England. She talked about the delights of having their own special 'White Train' to take them to the many places of interest they visited, of the warmth of the sea and the beauty of our beaches, and the excitement of a safari in the Kruger National Park. Clearly she loved talking about it to someone who knew the country and the time sped by very agreeably. Intermittently I could not help noticing how she surreptitiously passed morsels of food to the Corgis sitting quietly at her feet. After lunch we withdrew to another room where we were able to mix with the other guests over coffee, and then after she had departed with Princess Alexandra we were promptly ushered out of the Palace. Altogether a most memorable occasion and when, only a few years ago, I came across a copy in my possession of the formal publication celebrating the Royal Visit to South Africa of 1947, it contained so many happy photographs of her with her family that I decided to send it to her as a small gift and received a kind acknowledgement via her private secretary.

Private Practice at the Wellington Hospital
When in 1973 I was appointed to Papworth and Addenbrooke's Hospitals, Ben Milstein told me that he did not engage in private practice and so I agreed that at least for the first few years neither would I. At that time the starting salary of a full-time consultant in the NHS was not generous and I can remember how, with wry amusement, I learned that our senior registrar's salary, with the extra-duty payments that he earned, was significantly higher than mine. However, we had enough to live on to start with and it was only when the school bills started to come in that things became tight. As the decade progressed and I became more established I recognised that there was an opportunity for a small amount of private practice in cardiac surgery in East Anglia. So I changed my contract to nine-elevenths (9/11) of the full-time salary in order to allow

me to do a limited amount of private work if such existed. At first this was indeed limited but was later helped by a few rich Greek referrals from John Kapetenakis, who had returned to Rhodes after training in cardiology at Papworth. I also developed a small East African Indian practice through connections with a physician in Peterborough. However this was done more on a charitable basis and both the hospital and I charged significantly less than was the usual fee.

Then sometime during early 1981 I received a call from Dr Arthur Levin asking me to see him at the Wellington Hospital in London. Arthur had been associated with the Wellington when it was owned by The British and Commonwealth Shipping Company and had stayed on as Medical Director after the hospital had been bought by Humana in 1977. They were now in the process of expanding the facility by building an additional 110- bed hospital close to the original one. When we met, he presented a rather grandiose scheme in which he suggested that the whole of the new hospital might be devoted to cardiovascular medicine and surgery and, unlike any other private hospital in England, it would then develop academic training programmes of sufficient quality to be approved by the Colleges for postgraduate training of junior staff. He went on to ask whether I would be prepared to become Director of such a project, with a handsome salary from Humana with whom he had already had preliminary discussions. Although in some ways it was an attractive challenge, I felt too committed to developing the transplant programme at Papworth to consider a return to London. Furthermore, our family had settled in so well that I could see no good reason for leaving Cambridge. There the matter rested until June 1982 when I began to operate on the occasional private patient at the Wellington when their convenience and that of the referring cardiologist dictated this. Initially I had anaesthetic help from my friend from Guy's days, John Simpson. Both he, and later Mike Thomson, proved to be a great help, not only with the anaesthesia but also with postoperative care and supervision in the days following the operation. I normally operated at Papworth all day Monday, Wednesday and Friday morning with Thursday given to ward rounds and administration and a clinic at Addenbrooke's on Friday afternoon. So I chose Tuesday for the Wellington. John Wallwork had started at Papworth in November 1981 and I thought it important that we should form a partnership for the practice in London. This would mean that either of us would be free to deal with an emergency in London or a transplant at Papworth if we were in the other place. Also, by sharing the income, there could be no resentment on John's part that I was away earning money in London while he was left to look after Papworth with Ben Milstein. This arrangement, whereby two consultants operated together on private patients, was regarded as being most unusual by our colleagues in London. However, it worked well for us and I soon augmented the team by engaging the help of Paul Curry, who provided a superb cardiological service throughout the years that followed. The practice grew quite rapidly so that I felt the need to buy a small apartment near the Wellington. This meant that I was able to drive to London on Monday evening, see the patients who were to be operated on the next day, and then retire to the flat for a night's rest. John preferred to drive down early Tuesday morning.

Towards the end of the year Arthur Levin approached me again, this time with a different plan. He wanted to increase the throughput of cardiac surgery in the hospital and had learned that German patients had the right to ask to be referred abroad if they had to wait longer than three months for their surgery in Germany. Some were being sent to private hospitals in America and Arthur thought there was a potential to attract patients to the fine facilities that the Wellington offered, and that they would find London more convenient than Houston where many were going. He had already made contact with a man called Rheinhart Fischer who had been involved with such referrals and his suggestion was that Rheinhart should take me to a number of specified German hospitals, where I would talk to the relevant cardiologists and try to interest them in sending patients to the Wellington. Given my involvement with the UK Cardiac Surgical Register I could show them how our results compared with the national norms, and also take the opportunity of reviewing specific cases with them. I thought that this scheme might be worth exploring and so agreed to it but on the clear understanding that John and I would still only be able to operate at the Wellington on Tuesdays, where we would need to have access to two operating theatres all day. On this basis Arthur appointed me Director of Cardiac Surgical Services at the Wellington with a retainer of £1,000 per month.

During the next few months I made several weekend visits to Germany when I would be collected by Rheinhart and taken to meet cardiologists at hospitals that he had planned for me. I was always received politely and although the majority showed little interest there were some who were enthusiastic enough to agree to refer patients on a trial basis. So we arranged a schedule whereby the patient and one relative would be flown to London and admitted to the Wellington on a Sunday. I would see them with an interpreter on Monday evening and, having reviewed their notes and Xrays, get their consent for operation the following morning. I explained that both John Wallwork and I would be operating on them and that after we had returned to Cambridge on Tuesday evening their postoperative management would be in the hands of our anaesthetist and cardiologist whom they would have already met. I also stressed that we had a surgical assistant living in the hospital and that if there was any need for a surgical intervention one or other of us would always be available to return and deal with this. We would see them again in a week's time and if all were well the hospital would arrange for their transfer back to Germany at the weekend when, as was the practice in Germany, they would be sent to a rehabilitation centre for four to six weeks. This was a luxury not then available to British patients.

Having received the first patients in June 1983, the referrals were slow to start with. However, the feedback from patients to their German cardiologists must have been positive because the numbers increased steadily and we also began to get referrals from new cardiologists. By the beginning of 1984 we were often operating on three or four German patients each week and later in the year the demand became more than we could cope with. The other cardiac surgeons who used the Wellington, some of whom I knew well, had initially viewed our activity with a degree of scepticism but I was now able to reverse this by inviting them to participate in the programme so that by July 1989, when I became President of the Royal College of Surgeons and stopped operating at the Wellington, we were treating between five and six hundred patients per year. As can be imagined, this was also much to the satisfaction of the Wellington and its owners Humana, so I felt I had repaid in part their previous generosity in funding the artificial heart work.

The Stress begins to tell

The intensity of my surgical work and other commitments increased throughout the 1980s. I began to sleep badly and became increasingly troubled by symptoms that I ascribed to a probable duodenal ulcer. An example of the sort of life I was leading was recorded during a week in May 1987:

Friday 15. Consulted GP because of increasing severity of indigestion, precipitated chiefly by tiredness. Then on to transplant at Papworth returning at 3am.

Saturday 16. Worked at Papworth until 2.30 pm. Then saw Ann off to London as too exhausted to accompany her to dinner with friends as planned.

Sunday 17. Worked at home in morning preparing lecture for Brompton. Drove to London 2 pm; brief lunch with Ann in the flat and then on to Cowdray Park in Sussex to join in prize-giving at end of PRO-AM Golf Tournament in aid of Papworth Transplants. Returned home by 11.45 pm.

Monday 18. Heart-lung meeting at 8am. Operated all day, returning by 8.30 pm.

Tuesday 19. Operated first at Addenbrooke's at 8am. Then drove to London and operating at Wellington by 11.30 am. Across town to Brompton for 2pm lecture and stayed for discussion until 3.30 pm. Then to College of Surgeons by 4pm for meeting of the Court of Examiners with the President. Back to the Wellington and then to the Brompton for the Official Dinner. Returned to sleep at flat by 11pm.

Wednesday 20. Meeting with Ron Hytof (Chief Executive of Wellington) re. German Private Practice at 9am. To College of Surgeons by 11am for quarterly meeting of Regional Advisers and Tutors. Depart early at 12.15 to get to Paddington by 1.50 pm to address monthly meeting of Chairmen of Regional Health Authorities on "Cardiac Surgery and Cardiac Transplantation". Then to General Medical Council for 6 monthly meeting; left early in order to keep dental appointment at 5pm in Marylebone. Then across London to Great Ormond Street Hospital (by which time severe indigestion, needing milk) to see 14 year old boy with Cardiologists and Marc de Leval. Having assessed, then talk to parents about transplantation and then on to the GMC dinner at Apothecaries Hall.

Thursday 21. See patients at Wellington early and then on to the GMC for rest of Council meeting. Leave early to present data on Regional Distribution of Cardiac Surgery in UK to Working Party of the British Cardiac Society meeting at John Parker's rooms in Wimpole Street. Leave before meeting completed in order to return to flat, bath, pick up Ann and then go to the Savoy for the Wellington Charity Ball. Ann drives back to Cambridge (slowly) arriving back at 2 am.

Friday 22. Operate at Papworth in morning; lunchtime consultation at Evelyn Hospital; clinic at Addenbrooke's; home by 6.45 pm. Get cross (unreasonably) with Ann because I haven't eaten all day and supper is delayed.

Saturday morning. Present Grand Rounds at Addenbrooke's – and so it goes on ………… I begin to feel immensely weary at times and as if I am burning myself out.

But I was now on a roller-coaster and although I knew I ought to shed some of my activities I couldn't decide which. Perhaps the most obvious was to give up private practice at the Wellington. However I was reluctant to do without the financial independence that this afforded and ended up carrying on as before. In July I had a wonderful holiday in Southern Africa with William, who was then just sixteen. We went first to Natal and Zululand and then to a number of game camps surrounding and within the Okavango Delta in Botswana. This is one of the wonders of Africa that I had always wanted to see. The Okavango River rises in Angola and then crosses into Botswana where, instead of turning west to empty into the Atlantic it goes east and ends up in an inland delta in an arid part of northern Botswana. The annual flooding of the delta, which takes place during July and August, results in a great migration of every kind of animal towards the delta and its surrounds, making for some of the best game viewing in the world. This was a very special holiday for William and me and I returned to work feeling mightily refreshed.

However, the pressure continued and was perhaps responsible for another memorable event that occurred in March 1988. About nine months earlier I had accepted an invitation to deliver the prestigious 1988 Upjohn Lecture at the Royal Society and had chosen for my title: "Heart transplantation and the National Health Service - A question of priorities". However, as time flashed by and my lecture remained unwritten, I regretted bitterly having done so. And then about two months before the due date I had a terrible nightmare in which I arrived at the lecture and found I had left my slides behind and also that I had no manuscript. As the minutes ticked by I could hear the audience becoming impatient and restless but simply could not face them. This dream stimulated me to get on with the preparation of the lecture, which I duly completed to my satisfaction. On the day of the lecture I arrived at the Royal Society in good time to get to know the hall and to run through my slides that I had spent many hours preparing. To my horror, when I opened my briefcase, I found that the slide case I had brought contained not the carefully prepared slides for my lecture but ones from a lecture I had delivered at Brunel University the previous November. It was just like my nightmare. And when the projectionist asked me what I was going to do I replied that I thought I would simply go home! However, somehow I retained a modicum of wit. I duly started the lecture normally and then when it came to where I would have shown my first slide, I explained what had happened and proceeded to deliver my prepared text. I seemed to be able to take the audience with me and despite going on for too long the response afterwards was gratifying. Indeed, some were kind enough to say that the lecture had been interesting enough not to have depended on slides!

By the middle of 1988 my bouts of indigestion had increased to the extent that my GP referred me to John Hunter, a gastroenterologist at Addenbrooke's. He was initially doubtful that my symptoms were arising from the gut but an endoscopy revealed two active duodenal ulcers and I was put on appropriate treatment with the assurance that this would resolve matters. However, despite repeated courses of treatment I continued to suffer from bouts of severe indigestion after periods of stress and insomnia. Eventually by early December and after a further endoscopy, John Hunter decided that the only way of giving medical treatment a chance of healing the ulcer would be for me to take a complete rest from work for two or three months. Once this decision had been made, my colleagues at Papworth and the management of the hospital reacted sympathetically and Steve Large, our experienced and very able Senior Registrar, was appointed locum consultant and took over my duties. I was able to enjoy a fortnight's skiing with the children after Christmas and decided to take a holiday in South Africa with Ann during the latter part of January. Just before leaving, on 15th January 1989, I recorded the following in my journal: "Ten years yesterday since the first transplant at Papworth. Who could have thought then that all the rest would follow."

Ann and I enjoyed a wonderful three-week holiday in South Africa. We spent most of the time in the Cape at Tom's farm near Plettenberg Bay. This of course was where we had first met and I loved being able to enjoy again the beauty of the beaches and the sea, and the walks on Robberg which I had got to know so well. It also gave me time to think about my health and future activities. I now realised quite clearly that my duodenal ulcer and chronic insomnia were inter-related and that both were a reflection of the overwork and stress I had subjected myself to during the previous decade. However, with rest, good food, a chance to read and regular nights my insomnia and ulcer symptoms improved. In February I enjoyed a pleasant trip to Western Canada during which I was Visiting Professor at Edmonton and then went to Lake Louise that I had last visited 34 years earlier during my first working summer in Canada before embarking on my career in medicine.

When I resumed work in March I felt fully fit and my sleep pattern was much improved. I resolved to lead a more regular life with more time at home over the weekends and fewer external distractions. I was also conscious that there was a possibility that I might soon be elected President of the Royal College of Surgeons and that if this occurred I would certainly have to give up private practice at the Wellington with the heavy demands that this was making on my life. On 21st March I heard with great pleasure that Margaret Turner-Warwick had been elected President of the Royal College of Physicians, the first woman to be so honoured and one that I considered would be amongst the best that the College would ever be likely to have. Then at the end of Council on 13th April I was elected President of the Royal College of Surgeons of England. It was both wonderful and humbling to receive the congratulations of my colleagues at the Council Club dinner that evening. As it turned out, the Chairman that night was Ian (later Lord) McColl, who had asked me to introduce him. This was a special pleasure as Ian, who is a few months younger than me, had taught me Physiology at Guy's when I was a 2nd MB student and he a demonstrator in the Department of Physiology, whilst studying for his Primary FRCS examination. I admired his integrity and his subsequent achievements as Professor of Surgery at Guy's and had encouraged him to stand for Council.

The next three months were spent preparing for the Presidency. I gave up the Wellington practice and re-arranged my duties at Papworth so that I would continue to operate all day Monday and Friday morning, retaining my clinic at Addenbrooke's on Friday afternoon. This would leave me free to be in London during the middle of the week. I handed over the Transplant Programme to John Wallwork and the hospital advertised and then appointed Steve Large to a substantive consultant post. I also gave up the various administrative duties that I had been responsible for. In all this I received great consideration from the Chief Executive of the hospital, Stephen Bridge, who willingly helped to facilitate these arrangement so that by the time I was admitted to the Presidency as the first item on the agenda at the Meeting on 13th July I felt prepared for the challenge. Thus began one of the most interesting and satisfying periods of my life.

Chapter 7
Presidency of the Royal College of Surgeons (1989-1992)

My election to the Presidency of the Royal College of Surgeons of England was one of the proudest occasions of my life, and one of which I could not help wishing my dear mother could have been aware. After my father's early death, her world had largely been centred around giving Elizabeth and me the best possible start to life, not only with respect to our education but also with wanting to imbue in us the personal standards and principles which she held so dear. She had seen my 'wobble' when, after having decided to change from engineering, I withdrew from medical school and returned to mining exploration in Canada. Thankfully, she had also lived just long enough to see my return to Guy's and know that I was firmly committed to medicine. Throughout my life I have always felt that I owe her so much of whatever success I have achieved and only wish that she might have lived longer to share some of it.

Medical royal colleges have different statutes and rules with respect to the election of their presidents. The Physicians elect theirs by the Fellows who had to come to London on a prescribed day to vote in person at the College. With us, the Fellows of the College elect the Council and then Council elects the President. This is conducted by secret ballot at the end of the April meeting. The Secretary of the College distributes a list of current members eligible for election excluding only those whose term on Council will finish in July and the retiring President Each member then places a cross against the name of his or her preferred candidate, after which the voting papers are collected by the Secretary in a box and then, having returned to his table, he reads out the names one by one. In order to be elected, the President has to achieve a simple majority of those present and voting, and successive ballots are held until this happens. Three years previously Ian Todd and I had tied with an equal number of votes and he had been elected by virtue of his seniority on fellowship. This had been much to my relief as I certainly did not feel ready for the job. However, on this occasion my election was achieved with a substantial majority on the second ballot and it was reassuring to know that I would start with this degree of support from my Council.

The next three months prior to taking up office was a busy time. As mentioned, I gave up my practice at the Wellington Hospital but still had full duties at Papworth to compete with preparations for the task ahead. I also had to respond to over 200 letters of congratulation from friends and colleagues, the content of some of which I found quite overwhelming. Many surgeons were pleased to know that the balance had shifted from London to the Regions and also that although I would be representing surgery as a whole, I came from one of the smaller specialties, most presidents in the past having been general surgeons. The fact that at 56 I was the youngest President-elect on record was also well received.

Visiting the Past Presidents

I decided that it would be both polite and valuable to visit the four living Past Presidents. Of these Lord (Arthur) Porritt was the most senior, having been President twenty six years earlier (1960-1963), after which he became the first New Zealander to be Governor General of his country. He had also been a great athlete, having come third in the 100 metres at the Olympic Games in 1924. Ever since then, except for the war years, he and Harold Abrahams, who had won the race, used to dine with their wives on its anniversary. When they came to make the film "Chariots of Fire", Arthur told them he didn't think making a film about a race would work and would not allow his name to be used by whoever was to act his part. After the great success of "Chariots of Fire" he admitted that he rather regretted this! I got to know him after I joined Council and had huge admiration for him. He had great natural charm and was a born leader. When we met after my election he stressed that it was Council's responsibility to take tough decisions and gave me advice on how best to achieve this. He backed this up with his unqualified support throughout my Presidency.

I knew Lord (Rodney) Smith less well. Since demitting office he had been active in the House of Lords and had diminished his association with the College. When Ann and I went to see him and his wife Sue at their house in Marlow we were graciously received. He had been a strong and successful President (1973-1977) and again was able to offer much useful advice. He emphasised the distinctive roles of the BMA (British Medical Association) and the Medical Royal Colleges, in which the former is primarily responsible for the interests of doctors whereas the latter have as their chief aim education, training and protection of standards for the benefit of patients. He spoke of the importance of the 'Conference of Medical Royal Colleges' which he had helped found as an instrument for achieving unity of purpose amongst the colleges. As far as the Presidency was concerned he reflected his own rather autocratic style, believing that one should listen to advice but not commit yourself until you had come to your own judgement and then stick with it. He advised against allowing agenda items to go to the vote unless absolutely necessary.

Some days later I was surprised to receive a 6-page letter from him concerning events surrounding the election of his successor, Reginald Murley. He said he thought this was sometimes still talked about and wanted to put the record straight. This related to a difficult time when a small number of Council members tried to get Rodney to remain President for an additional year. Owing to the death in office of his predecessor, Edward Muir, he had already served three years and nine months and a further extension was clearly against the rules as they then were and still are. The division within Council persisted right up to the day of election and this became a protracted and difficult event, which of course Rodney had to chair. However, good practice prevailed and Reggie Murley, much to his surprise, was eventually elected President. I was only aware of the rough outline of what had happened twelve years earlier and was able to reassure Rodney that the matter was no longer an issue of contention and indeed that it was very rarely, if ever, referred to. I did however feel that as a matter of historical interest and accuracy I should show his letter to Reggie Murley and then to Ronald Johnson-Gilbert, who as Secretary at the time was responsible for the process of the election, and after receiving their comments I placed all the correspondence in the confidential archives of the College.

Reggie, as he was always known by his wide circle of friends, was a very different person from his two predecessors. When I joined Council he still had one year to serve on it after relinquishing the Presidency and it was during this time that our friendship began. Indeed he adopted me as his "nephew-in-law" as his wife Daphne was the cousin of Betty Lund, Uncle

Max's wife. He was a man of great exuberance and vitality who always spoke his mind directly and with the utmost clarity. His extraordinary memory for people and events formed the basis for his fund of stories and on social occasions laughter was generally loudest in whatever part of the room he was sitting. Later, when I became President, he frequently telephoned me on a Sunday evening to give me his views on what was happening in the world of surgery and how the College should react to these events. He was at that time Chairman of the Hunterian Trustees and before I started in office he insisted on taking me to Westminster Abbey to view John Hunter's tomb and to tell me about the life of his hero. This included how, during the previous century, Hunter's body had been removed from the crypt of St Martin's in the Fields and re-interred in the Abbey. He decided we should walk from the College to Westminster and on the way I could not help noticing that he was taking frequent tablets of glycerine trinitrate, which is a drug to relieve angina. I asked him whether he had consulted a cardiologist about his heart disease and he confirmed that he had, and mentioned the name of an elderly retired man that I knew. I suggested he should perhaps seek the opinion of a more modern cardiologist and then heard nothing more until nine months later when I received a call from him from the Wellington Hospital. He announced he had eventually taken my advice and having been appropriately investigated was about to undergo cardiac surgery the next morning and that Gareth Rees was to perform the operation. I said I was relieved it was going to be dealt with and wished him a speedy recovery, to which he replied: "You know dear boy, I really wanted you to operate on me, but then I thought if I perished it would be bad for your Presidency". What greater consideration could I have been shown!

Sir Alan Parks succeeded Reggie Murley and when he died in office Geoffrey Slaney was elected. I was on Council by that time and came to admire his good judgement during the three years of his Presidency. He was a fine leader and had been widely respected during his time as Barling Professor of Surgery in Birmingham, where he built up an excellent academic department with a reputation for turning out well-trained surgeons. He, like Alan Parks, was much respected by the Presidents of the other surgical colleges, both in Britain and abroad, and did a lot towards strengthening relationships between colleges. His impact on the affairs and fortunes of the Royal College of Surgeons of England was considerable and he and his charming wife, Jo, did much to enhance the social life of the College.

Priorities and early activities

Driving back from my visit to see Geoff in Birmingham in May, I realised that in some respects I was reasonably well prepared to take on the Presidency. Six years accompanying first Alan Parks and then Geoff Slaney as a member of the quarterly "Joint Meetings of Surgical Colleges" had given me a feel for intercollegiate affairs as well as a good understanding of the position with respect to the Intercollegiate Specialty Fellowship examinations and the need for revising the existing FRCS exam. An equivalent time on the General Medical Council had provided an insight into disciplinary and educational issues facing the medical profession that I could never otherwise have obtained. I also had some knowledge of how the Department of Health worked as a result of my encounters with it over the transplant programme at Papworth. Furthermore, I had acquired some experience of how surgery was organised in other countries – particularly the United States and Europe – as a result of my travels associated with transplantation. But there were still requirements for the job that I felt uncertain about. These included the ceremonial and speech-making demands, which I approached with more than a little apprehension.

I decided it would be useful to draw up a list of preliminary objectives and priorities before I started. I accepted these might need to be adapted in the light of experience but believed that some specific tasks needed to be addressed. They were recorded as follows:

1. Restore morale on Council and make the College more relevant to its Fellows.

2. Form a closer relationship with the Surgical Specialty Associations and keep the Anaesthetists and Dental Surgeons within the College.

3. Secure better countrywide training and career structure for young surgeons.

4. Achieve an appropriate title for the revised FRCS and get more candidates to take our exam.

5. Expand consultant surgical numbers.

6. Work towards the introduction of an indicative Specialist Register and then periodic recertification for those on it.

7. Get a successful £10 million Appeal going.

8. Place the Hunterian Institute on a sound financial basis. (Partly dependent on 7.)

Looking back on these, I see that most were achieved, though some such as an indicative Specialist Register only came many years later. However, some were not and as will be seen the Anaesthetists left Lincoln's Inn Fields soon after I took office to start their own College. I also had a lot of difficulty with the Appeal, which only really got going during my last year, and the Hunterian Institute was finally closed down to make space for the College to become a centre for surgical training rather than research.

I also wanted to introduce an open style of Presidency and be more accessible both to those working within the College and to the Fellowship at large, particularly those who served the College such as our Regional Advisers and Tutors. As part of getting to know the latter and meet more Fellows up and down the country, I decided that during the first six months I would visit each of the thirteen Health Regions and hold afternoon meetings with the local Fellows, during which I would hear their views and answer questions as to what the College was doing about some of the problems they were facing. These proved to be most informative and because I was still in active surgical practice I believe I carried more credibility with Fellows than if I had been retired.

With regard to chairing Council, I came across somewhere – I know not where – the following "Rules for the Appointment of Speaker of the House of Commons" and thought they might be applicable to this task:

1. Imperturbable good temper, tact and patience.

2. Previous legal training if possible.

3. The possession of innate gentlemanly feelings; which involuntarily command respect and deference.

4. Personal dignity in voice and manner.

I doubt that I lived up to these ideals but may have done better than Michael Martin who was forced to resign from the office of Speaker in June 2009!

I was duly admitted to the Presidency at the Council meeting on 13th July 1989 as the second item of formal business. Ian Todd handed over the Presidential badge of office and the gown that went with it and I then chaired the rest of the proceedings. Ann and I now moved into the very pleasant President's Lodge, which is situated within Nuffield College This was immediately adjacent to and connected with my office in the main building and made for efficient working when I was in London. Our future routine became that Ann and I drove to London on Monday evening after supper following my day's operating at Papworth. I then had all Tuesday, Wednesday and Thursday for College business, before returning to Cambridge on either Thursday evening or early Friday morning for my operating list at Papworth and then a clinic at Addenbrooke's Hospital in the afternoon.

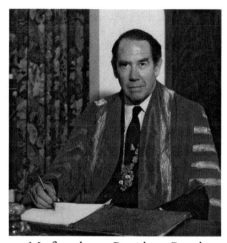

My first day as President, Royal College of Surgeons of England.

The Lodge was comfortable and a good place for entertaining. Ann enjoyed her days in London and soon got to know the Porters, telephonists, catering and other

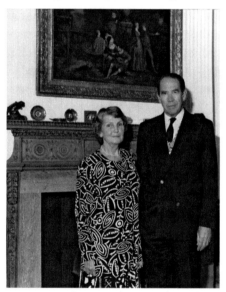

Ann and me in the Presidential Lodge, RCS.

staff who worked in the building. They appreciated her interest and with our many social occasions she led a busy life and soon came to enjoy her new role in the College. Indeed, she remarked later that it had been one of the happiest times of our marriage.

My life soon became very busy. I inherited an efficient Secretary, Alison Elliot, who had already served my three predecessors. Her habit was to get rid of all the previous President's correspondence when his successor took over, which I found occasionally made for difficulties. So we came to an arrangement whereby my personal correspondence was retained separate from official business, with the latter being kept on file for future reference. Within the first few weeks I was invited to meetings with the Chief Medical Officer, Sir Donald Acheson, who gave me lunch at the Athenaeum, and with the Secretary of State for Health, Virginia Bottomley, at Richmond House. The White Paper outlining the Conservative Government's proposed reforms for the National Health Service had been published a few months earlier and had caused considerable concern amongst the medical profession. In essence, Margaret Thatcher believed that the NHS was under-managed and also that it would be more efficient if there were a stronger competitive element in the provision of Health Care. This led to the attempt to create an artificial market within hospitals and General Practice. The latter were to be given the option of becoming 'Fund-holders', whereby they would become small businesses purchasing care for their patients from various 'providers', mainly the hospitals. And the hospital sector would be divided into commissioners and providers. The idea here was that the freedom given to commissioners to purchase care from whom they chose would stimulate competition amongst the providers and hence increase efficiency.

Many of us had serious concerns about the wisdom of these proposals. I had personal doubts about the substantial bureaucracy needed for such an artificial market within the setting of the NHS. I also believed that the spirit of public service, which was so strong a feature amongst those who worked for the National Health Service, would be jeopardised by the introduction of these reforms. The White Paper was put out to consultation and received many hours of attention and debate from the British Medical Association and all the Medical Royal Colleges, and our responses contained some sensible recommendations. However, before the NHS Reform Bill passed through Parliament, Kenneth Clarke replaced Virginia as Secretary of State as Secretary of State and very few of these were incorporated. Interestingly, the Labour Party who at the time opposed the reforms vigorously, retained most of them when they came to power six years later.

The Anaesthetists depart the College
Another issue that occupied much of my time during the first few months was the separation of the Anaesthetists from our College. A Faculty of Anaesthetists had been formed within the College in 1948, one year after

a similar Faculty of Dental Surgeons. The Boards of each Faculty were elected by their Fellows, and the Dean and Vice Dean, who were elected by each Board, sat on the Council of the College of Surgeons. Anaesthetics had become a rapidly expanding specialty and by the early 1980s there were those amongst them who thought the time had come to establish their own college. Others, however, were content with the existing situation and saw advantages in remaining within the accommodation provided by the Royal College of Surgeons (RCS). As a result of discussions within the specialty and much debate in Council an arrangement was arrived at in 1986 whereby the Anaesthetists were given the status of "The College of Anaesthetists" within the RCS with their own President and with more or less complete independence. Dr Aileen Adams was elected the first President, with whom we had excellent relations. Shortly before I became President, Michael Rosen was elected her successor and then, within a fortnight of my taking office, he came to tell me that the Anaesthetists wished to separate from us completely. One reason for their desire to become wholly independent was that in due course they would be able to gain the title of "Royal College of Anaesthetists", which was otherwise denied them so long as they remained a College within our Royal College. I could understand their aspirations and determined to work towards an amicable separation. However, some of my Council were not pleased and there was understandable criticism that we had recently gone through much trouble to give them their current status only to find that this was not sufficient. It was also felt strongly that the complete separation which they now sought was not consistent with them remaining in their present accommodation. So in due course they moved out, thankfully with good relations having been preserved, and four or five years later they achieved the Royal prerogative and acquired a fine building of their own.

College visits abroad

Unlike the Edinburgh College of Surgeons, who made regular visits abroad to hold joint meetings with other surgical groups and colleges, we had neglected this. I saw the value of such visits and was fortunate during my Presidency in being able to lead two College visits abroad that were very well attended. The first of these took place in early October 1989 when we held joint meetings, first with the Royal College of Surgeons of Thailand and then with the Academies of Medicine of Malaysia and Singapore. I had previously met the Queen of Thailand when I delivered the 2nd Kitiyakara Lecture in Bangkok in September 1988. This was in honour of the Queen's brother who had been a cardiac surgeon and who had done some of his training with Lord Brock at Guy's Hospital. On this later visit, accompanied by some sixty Fellows and their spouses, we had a royal reception at the Palace, where we were graciously received by the King and Queen and with whom we exchanged gifts.

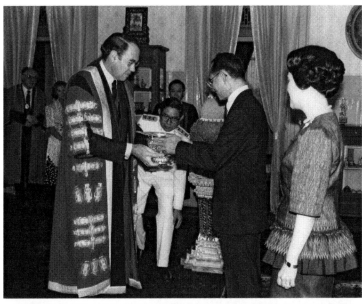

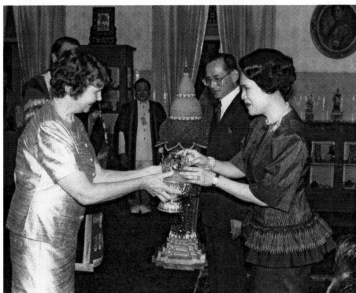

Ann and me exchanging gifts with the King and Queen of Thailand

Two years later I was I was privileged to receive an Honorary Fellowship from the Royal College of Surgeons of Thailand, awarded to me by the King's daughter, Princess Sirindhorn.

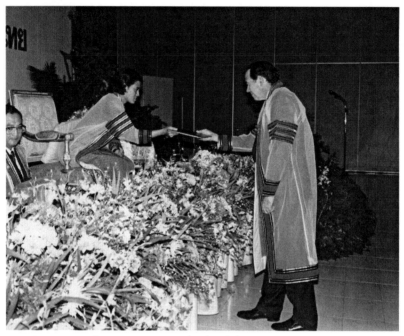

Receiving the Hon. FRCS Thailand from Princess Sirindhorn

Our Thai hosts were most hospitable, the joint scientific meeting went well and it was altogether a most worthwhile and enjoyable visit. Then it was on to Kuala Lumpur for the 23rd Malaysia and Singapore Congress of Medicine. This was organised by the Academy of Medicine of Malaysia and the King of Malaysia attended the opening ceremony. He had graduated in Law from Nottingham University and gave an excellent opening address on "Law and Medical Ethics". (Ten years later I had the pleasure of giving his citation when he was made an Honorary FRCS England) I had decided to respond with the introduction of my speech in Bahasa Malaysia and sought the help of one of the local secretaries to translate what I wanted to say and then practised it phonetically beforehand. This proved to be much appreciated by the audience. Again there was lots of hospitality to be enjoyed and we returned to England sufficiently convinced of the value of such visits that we set about organising the next one to Pakistan and India two years later.

This took place in October 1991 and again was heavily subscribed to by Council members and Fellows from as far afield as Australia, New Zealand, the United States, Malta and Canada. We went first to Karachi where we held a joint meeting with the College of Physicians and Surgeons of Pakistan. I made the opening address and also gave a lecture on "Thoughts on the Present, Past and Future of Cardiac Surgery", and at the end of the meeting was made an Honorary Fellow of their College. Before moving on to India, some of us accepted an invitation to Peshawar, capital of the North West Frontier Province, by Mohammad Kabir, Professor of Surgery at the Khyber Medical College and Principal of the Lady Reading Hospital. Kabir had spent five years training in surgery in England during the early 1960s and had become highly respected in Peshawar, where he was a good friend of the Governor's and later became Secretary of Health for the Frontier Province.

On our first evening in Peshawar, Ann and I were invited to dinner at his home. However, she was unwell and I went alone. There followed one of those memorable but rare occasions when you meet someone and soon know that you have formed the basis of a deep and lasting friendship. We kept in touch over the years during which I made several more trips to Peshawar, always being a guest in his large home that also provided for many relations besides his immediate family. On one of these visits I was taken on a surgical ward-round by one of his senior residents. After seeing a number of patients we came to a young man in a bed who was declared to be an "SBI". I didn't know what an SBI was, but not wishing to display my ignorance said nothing and we moved on. However, by the time we came to the fifth SBI I felt I had to confess and ask what the diagnosis was. He laughed heartily and said: "Oh Sir, stray bullet injury, Sir". This reflected the custom of rifles being carried by a large proportion of the male population, which were often randomly fired into the air at times of celebration or excitement.

While in Peshawar during that first College visit, Kabir arranged for us to be taken up the Khyber Pass as far as the Afghanistan border. We were accompanied by a military escort and on the way back were entertained at the Khyber Rifles Mess. This was a most impressive building and contained photographs of many world leaders and famous people who had visited the Mess over the years. I also noticed that they had shields of various organisations on their walls, and on a return visit some years later I donated our Royal College of Surgeons shield to join these.

From Pakistan we went to Delhi for a joint meeting with the Association of Surgeons of India. We stayed at the rather grand Taj Palace Hotel and again there were receptions, opening ceremonies, and lectures to be given from both sides. We also had time to see some of the sights and explore the old city before it was time to return home. During my time at the College I made many other visits abroad, giving lectures and being a guest at meetings of other surgical colleges. These included trips to Zimbabwe, Toronto, San Francisco, South Africa, Australia (twice), Thailand and New Orleans. Surgeons on the whole are "clubbable" people and I was invariably met with kindness and hospitality.

The Royal Visit
I was fortunate in that some months before my Presidency started, plans had been made for Her Majesty the Queen, who was our Visitor and an Honorary Fellow, to visit the College. This took place on 21st November 1989 when she was accompanied by Prince Phillip, also an Honorary Fellow, and the Mayor of Westminster.

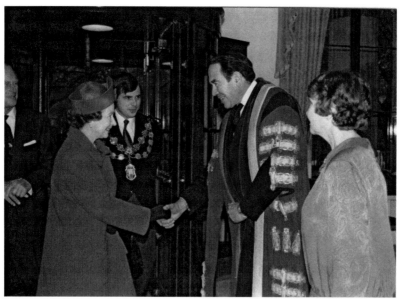

Receiving the Queen at the start of her visit to the RCS, November 1989

For her arrival I had arranged that Council members would stand in a large semicircle in the imposing entrance hall of the College. The Queen, however, had already had a demanding morning opening the new Session of Parliament, and having greeted her and seen what was in front of her she said: "I can't possibly say Hello to all these people". I reassured her this was not necessary but as we started to walk past the Council members she must have begun to feel guilty because she stopped in front of Professor John Blandy, who was a distinguished Urologist, and after being introduced asked what his specialty was. Back came the reply, "Waterworks Ma'am", and the conversation stopped there! However, she was delighted to meet Lord Porritt when she got to the Library. She knew him well because he was first made "Surgeon in Ordinary" to her parents, when they were Their Royal Highnesses the Duke and Duchess of York, and then later became Sergeant Surgeon to the Queen. Following his term as President of the College, he became her Governor General in New Zealand. After the Library she had a conducted tour of the Hunterian Museum by the Chairman of Trustees, Sir Reginald Murley, and then opened the new Hanson Suite for Surgical Training, funded by Lord Hanson, who was a Patron of the College. Her visit culminated in a grand Tea Party in the Lumley Hall during which she met more Fellows and members of

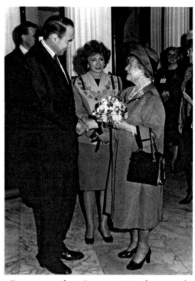

Greeting the Queen Mother with Dame Shirley Porter, Mayor of Westminster.

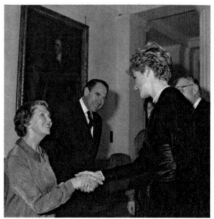

Ann greeting Princess Diana, RCS.

Staff. The next day I received a letter from her Private Secretary, Sir Robert Fellowes, saying how interesting she and the Duke had found the visit and how much they had enjoyed seeing so many old friends on their tour. I responded on behalf of Council and everyone associated with the College, and after thanking her and the Duke of Edinburgh most sincerely for having given so generously of their time concluded by saying, "It is an occasion that will be remembered by us all. You left behind a warm glow of pride and pleasure that will enhance the morale of the College for a long time to come." I was particularly fortunate in that during my time as President we had three other visits by Royalty to the College – the Queen Mother, Princess Ann and Princess Diana.

Besides visits overseas and Royal visits at home, there was much else to keep me busy. One of the attractions of the job was the range of issues one had to deal with and the variety of people one met. This is illustrated by notes made of some of the events during a week at the end of October 1989:

Saturday 28:   7.15 am left Reading following Council visit the previous day for 9am appointment in Cambridge. Papworth 10.30am to 1.30 pm. Then 6-7.15 pm Ann and I had drinks with Lord and Lady Rothschild at their home; both remarkable people.

Sunday 29:   Mainly devoted to preparing speech for GMC dinner and other College tasks for the coming week.

Monday 30:   Two difficult cases operated on at Papworth:

> (a) Redo ASD – entered right atrium on way in and had to do emergency cannulation and partial bypass before proceeding Happily ended alright.

> (b) Resection of aneurysm of ascending aorta and aortic valve replacement in 65 year old female. Good result. Left Papworth 6.15 pm for informal supper at Carlton Club at 7.45 with Secretary of State, Virginia Bottomley, and Sir Arnold Elton.

Tuesday 31:   College work and interviews in am. Lunch at GMC with Sir Robert Kilpatrick (President) and Peter Towers (Registrar).
pm Visit by Sir Robert Fellowes and John Haslam in preparation for the Queen's visit.
Evening: Dinner in Lodge for Donald and Dorothy Ross and Chris and Diana McGregor.

Wed 1 November   College business all day, including interviewing John West about failures in the Examinations Department.
Evening: GMC Council Dinner. Replied to toast on behalf of the Presidents of the Royal Colleges.

Thursday 2:   College business all day. Gordon Reeves, new editor of The Lancet, for lunch. Martin Taylor and Michael O'Shea of Hanson's plc to view recently completed Hanson's Suite. Quiet evening preparing for next day's business.

Friday 3:   Joint meeting of Surgical Colleges with me in the Chair, am. and early pm. Informal Regional Presidential visit to SW Thames: 4.45 – 7.15pm.
Supper with E and D (sister and brother-in-law) on way back to Cambridge. Home by midnight
I must try and preserve more of the weekends for relaxation and "thinking time".

The NHS Reforms and Politics

I have already mentioned how concerned the medical profession was about many aspects of the proposed NHS Reform Bill and in the first few months of 1990 I had several private meetings with Kenneth Clarke, Secretary of State for Health, about this. The first was arranged by a surgeon, Sir Arnold Elton, who was Chairman of the Conservative Medical Society, and it took place in a corridor in the House of Commons, adjoining the room in which the NHS Bill was being discussed at Committee Stage. My meeting arose as a result of a request to the medical royal colleges by the Labour Peer, Lord Ennals, to provide him with research evidence that could be used against the Bill as it passed through the Lords. I responded that I felt a more productive approach would be if we could get the Secretary of State to agree in principle to a professional evaluation of the consequences of the Bill and its more contentious impact on health care services and standards. This could then be used as a basis for discussion between the Department of Health, leaders of the medical profession, and possibly health economists. Arnold had relayed this message on to Kenneth Clarke who then asked to see me.

I think initially he saw this as an opportunity to improve relations with the profession and also perhaps avoid an untidy battle in the House of Lords. He said that he favoured establishing an advisory group that could give advice to Health Authorities on specific issues related to the Bill after it had become law. I replied that I thought this was something that might grow out of a research evaluation but should not precede it. And I went on to suggest that time was of the essence and if he wanted the initiative to be seen as coming from him, then a statement by the Chief Medical

Officer at the Joint Consultants Committee meeting the next week was a good opportunity; otherwise it might look as if he was reacting to a threat of action from the House of Lords to coerce him into accepting a research evaluation of the Bill. He said he would think about this.

Finally, I said that I felt the BMA would have to be included as participants in the project. This he did not like. He didn't want a proposal like this to be used as yet another negotiating forum, and went on to mention that during his long life in politics Tony Grabham, who was then Chairman of Council of the BMA, was amongst the cleverest and most difficult negotiator he had ever come across. However, I replied that if the BMA were not included, it would look as if he was trying to split the profession and this would not be well accepted. Rather, I urged him to be "bold and optimistic".

Well, we did not get our evaluation of the potential consequences of the Bill. Instead we got a proposal from Ken Clarke for a 'Clinical Standards Advisory Group' (CSAG) to be included in the NHS Reform Act. This would be comprised of members recommended by the Conference of Medical Royal Colleges and it would have powers to investigate any aspect of the Health Service where there were concerns about a possible decline of standards as a result of introduction of the reforms. The problem here was that he wanted to specifically exclude the BMA from the Group. This was discussed by Conference of the Medical Royal Colleges who were generally in favour of the proposal. My own view, which I held particularly strongly, was that Tony Grabham, as current Chairman of Council of the BMA, had to be included. I wrote to Kenneth Clark twice about this, and on both occasions received a polite rejection. Some Presidents were prepared to meet him for further discussion but both Margaret Turner-Warwick and I saw his position as a blatant attempt to split the profession and devalue the importance of the BMA by implying that it had nothing to do with clinical standards. I went to see Sir George Godber, a much respected retired Chief Medical Officer for Health, for advice and his response was that if the Royal Colleges of Physicians and Surgeons did not participate in the discussions they were unlikely to get very far. So, after much deliberation, I decided not to go to the first meeting which took place between the Colleges and the Secretary of State, having made it clear to Kenneth Clarke that the Royal College of Surgeons could not be part of the CSAG unless the BMA were included. I was pleased subsequently by his concession at that meeting, to agree to include the Chairman of Council of the BMA in further discussions, and in the Statutory CSAG when it was enacted. I then felt happy to rejoin the talks and be as constructive as possible.

Junior Doctors' hours of work

Another political battle I had towards the end of my Presidency was with the Department of Health over the introduction of the 'New Deal on Junior Doctors Hours". This proposed that Junior Doctors should not work more than 72 hours per week. There was no doubt that many juniors were working far too hard and that this needed to be dealt with. However, as surgeons we had two concerns. We felt that a blanket imposition of 72 hours per week would result in many instances in a substitution of the rota system, in which a surgical team worked closely together, for shift working which would disrupt both training and continuity of care. We felt that with surgery being a craft specialty, in which exposure to technical experience was so important, training would inevitably be compromised by service demands if both were to be fitted into a 72 hour week.

Dr Diana Walford, as Deputy CMO, had the unenviable task of chairing the meetings about the New Deal that proved long and acrimonious. The BMA's Junior Committee, who to me always seemed to carry too much influence within the Council of the BMA, were absolutely committed to it. Most of the Royal Colleges were prepared to accept the change, although some like the Royal College of Physicians did so only with a degree of reluctance. However, I felt strongly that a degree of flexibility was needed for surgery if training and standards were not to suffer. I therefore proposed that surgical trainees who wished to be on duty for longer than 72 hours per week should be allowed to do so. I saw this applying particularly to more senior trainees who might of their own accord want to be present at interesting operations occurring outside their normal hours of duty. I stressed that they should not be put under pressure by their consultants to do this, and that their attendance should be voluntary and unpaid. Eventually, after much debate and to the relief of Dr Walford, the working group accepted this and the so-called 'English Clause' was incorporated in the final agreement. This worked well and I heard subsequently from both consultants and trainees how useful it had been in smoothing the transition to a much reduced working week. However, about six years later the Department of Health quietly abolished the Clause. Now, as I write, the European Working Time Directive has recently been introduced, reducing the hours to 48 per week. This, I believe, is having serious repercussions on both training and continuity of care and should never have been allowed to apply to the medical profession in Britain.

Demise of the Hunterian Institute

About the same time as the argument over the " New Deal on Junior Doctors Hours" was going on, I was having an internal battle with my Council. This was over the future of the Hunterian Institute where basic research was being pursued within the College. The background to this was that during Lord Brock's presidency he had been responsible for creating an Institute of Basic Medical Sciences. This was related to the extensive teaching of anatomy, physiology, biochemistry, pathology and pharmacology that was being given to trainee surgeons in preparation for the Primary FRCS examination. As teaching in the College declined, the departments turned more towards encouraging research in their respective subjects. This resulted in the Institute of Basic Medical Sciences being transformed into the Hunterian Institute, which initially received substantial financial support from London University. However, this was withdrawn in the early 1980s and the College then had to bear the full financial burden of the Institute, amounting to some £600,000 *per annum*. There was a perception amongst Council that research in some of the Departments was not of sufficient calibre to justify such a large expenditure. However, shortly before I became President, Sir Stanley Peart FRS was elected Master of the Hunterian Institute with a remit to improve research and concentrate this into one or two of the better departments if this was felt necessary. This indeed is what he achieved and by the mid-term of my Presidency we were left with a strong department in Pharmacology and a world-class research group in Magnetic Resonance Imaging that David Gaddian had brought with a team from Oxford.

Then in June 1991 there were calls for a special meeting of Council to review the future of the Hunterian Institute. In essence this arose from a powerful lobby within Council who wished to see the Institute closed down. Their argument was that we couldn't afford it and that in any case the College was not the right place for pursuing basic research and that the remaining groups were too small to be effective on their own. On the other hand I felt that we had given Stanley Peart a difficult task, in which he had largely succeeded, and that it would be seen as nothing short of betrayal by the Institute staff, who had already had many uncertainties and difficulties to deal with during the previous two years. Furthermore, I had made research in the Institute a central theme of many of my discussions with potential benefactors.

The special meeting was difficult, lasting nearly three hours, and with me very much in a minority. I did, however, manage to persuade the Council to accept a review of the activities of the Institute before coming to a decision to close it down. This would examine the pros and cons of continuing research in it and would have an external chairman. I also persuaded them not to predetermine the outcome of the review by dropping a resolution that funding of the Institute by the College should cease after June 1993. At the ensuing Council meeting, and after further discussion, it was agreed that a Working Party should be established to "review and advise on the balance, organisation and funding of teaching and research both within and without the College at Lincoln's Inn Fields." Five senior Council members were chosen to serve on this and I managed to persuade Sir Michael Peckham, who had recently retired as Chairman of the British Postgraduate Medical Federation, to be chairman. I also obtained the services of an independent secretary to the Working Party in the form of John Smith, a retired civil servant.

The Working Party met over a period of three months and published their report in the spring of 1992. It recommended closure of the Institute's research activities, whilst retaining teaching anatomy in the College. It also recommended the establishment of a Royal College of Surgeons surgical research fellowship scheme. These Fellowships would be the target for specific fund-raising and could be held in academic surgical units anywhere in England and Wales. It also advised that space vacated by the Institute research groups should be devoted to facilities for significantly expanding the number and variety of courses held in the College for surgical trainees.

Stan Peart remained loyal to the College to the end and before his departure managed to get the pharmacology group relocated at King's College, and David Gaddian's team at Great Ormond Street Hospital for Children, where they were very successful. Although, as can be seen, I was much opposed to the closure of the Hunterian Institute, I have to acknowledge that this was indeed the right decision. The research fellowship scheme has gone from strength to strength and the College attracts surgeons at all levels of their training to the fine courses and superb facilities that are now provided by the College

Social life at the College

Besides chairing Council and several other important committees, there were many social events related to the job. I presided at the major College Feasts, such as the Hunterian Banquet and the Buckston Browne Dinner, to which many of the 'great and the good' of the medical profession were invited. There were also many invitations from other colleges, specialist associations and livery companies to attend. I also had the responsibility of finding after-dinner speakers for the Quarterly Dinners, which were designed to attract Fellows and their spouses and friends to the College. Some of the most successful of these included Sir John Butterfield, Ludovic Kennedy, Michael O'Donnell, Jonathan Porritt, Brian Johnstone the great cricket commentator, and Cliff Morgan of Welsh rugby fame. The latter was a particularly happy occasion, with many of my old rugby friends amongst the guests. Lord Porritt was a regular attender of these dinners and when present I always placed him next to me. As soon as the Loyal Toast was given he would pull out a battered cigarette case and say "Have a cigarette, Terence". Although not a smoker, I always took one to keep him company and the two of us would sit puffing away at the top table, while I often endured severe looks from some of my colleagues. At the time, the Secretary was keen on turning the College into a non-smoking building but I resisted this in the knowledge that it would almost certainly reduce, if not entirely exclude, further visits by Arthur and his wife Kaye. I have already mentioned the Council Club Dinners and there was a very special one on 14th July 1990 to celebrate Arthur Porritt's 90th birthday. For me it was a golden evening and I felt there could not have been a more fitting climax to the end of my first year in office. I had the anxiety of introducing our illustrious Chairman but this went well and then Arthur spoke splendidly for 45 minutes without a note, at the end of which he kindly referred to a new phenomenon at the College that he called "The Terence Touch".

Another rather special occasion that took place at the end of the same year, was an appeal dinner I organised in honour of Tony Trafford. I had first known him and his wife Helen at Guy's when he was senior registrar and I houseman on the same medical firm. He had a razor-sharp mind and enormous capacity for hard work and later became a consultant physician at Brighton at the early age of 33. He also developed an interest in Conservative politics and was soon combining the difficult task of being an MP with a constituency in the Wrekin and a consultant practice

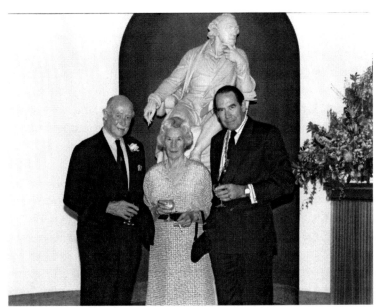

With Lord and Lady Porritt before his 90th birthday dinner, RCS.

on the South Coast. However, eventually he decided that his first love of medicine should prevail and he returned to the life of a full-time physician in Brighton.

He was involved with treating the victims of the Brighton bombing in 1984 and a knighthood followed. Then at the beginning of 1989 he was elected to the House of Lords as Minister of State for Health by Mrs Thatcher, and was subsequently entrusted with the task of seeing the NHS Reform Bill through the Upper House. It was at this time that I got to know him even better. He tackled the new task with his customary enthusiasm and went to great lengths to listen to the Presidents of most of the Royal Colleges and understand our concerns over some of the changes being proposed. He also helped to improve relations between Government and the BMA and it was a great shock and sense of loss to many when his commission came to such an abrupt and untimely end when he died at the early age of 57 in September 1989.

Some months after his death I was asked by Helen if I would become a Patron of the Trafford Appeal for Medical Research, which she had established as a memorial to Tony. I decided the best way I could contribute to the Appeal would be to hold a Dinner at the College of Surgeons, which would bring together his friends from politics, the medical profession, the Department of Health, the University of Sussex and other friends and colleagues from Guy's and Brighton. It was a grand evening and helped to raise a considerable sum of money. Apart from myself, I had planned for only two other speakers; Kenneth Clarke as Secretary of State for Health and Norman Tebbit who was also in the Cabinet, and who was once memorably described by Frank Johnson, the Parliamentary Sketchwriter, as "the Chingford Strangler". Besides being a political colleague, Tony had looked after Tebitt's wife when she sustained severe injuries as a result of the Brighton bombing and it was for this reason that I asked him to speak. About two weeks before the dinner, William Waldegrave took over from Kenneth Clarke as Secretary of State for Health. It was therefore agreed that he should speak instead of Clarke and I was pleased when he indicated he would like to use the occasion as an opportunity to present a more conciliatory approach to the medical profession. He did this extremely well despite the embarrassment of having Kenneth Clarke seated nearby, who I thought should have declined the invitation after he had demitted office. However, this was then spoiled by Tebbit's speech, most of which was good but which ended with some critical and unnecessary remarks about the medical profession and our resistance to the NHS Reform Bill. Not at all what I had wished for and regretted by many of those present, not least perhaps by William Waldegrave.

Another memorable, but entirely different occasion took place at the Austrian Embassy in September 1991at a lunch held in honour of the philosopher Karl Popper. Some years previously I had read most of "The Open Society and its Enemies" and although I did not understand all of it, I recognised him as one of the great philosophers of our age and was thrilled to meet him. After lunch we had the opportunity of a brief discussion during which I asked him why he had gone to New Zealand in 1936. He replied that he had offers from both Cambridge and New Zealand, which presented him with "an interesting moral dilemma". This resulted from his concern for a colleague in Austria, Freidrich Weissman, who was an enthusiastic follower of Ludwig Wittgenstein but who was "quite incapable of looking after himself". So he let him take the job in the philosophy department in Cambridge while he, Popper, went to New Zealand. He then added how when Weissman arrived in Cambridge Wittgenstein steadfastly avoided ever meeting him!

There were other more light-hearted social occasions, one of which was the annual cricket match played between members of Council and College staff. This was held on the cricket pitch in the lovely grounds of Down House, which had been Charles Darwin's home for most of his life and from where he had written "On the Origin of Species". It was situated near the village of Down in the beautiful Weald of Kent. After Darwin died his widow, Emma, continued to live in the house until her death in 1896. It was then used as a girls' school but in 1927 the surgeon George Buckston Browne bought it and presented it to the British Association for the Advancement of Science. Five years later he bought the surrounding 13 acres to establish a Surgical and Biological Research Institute. This was to be owned and run by the Royal College of Surgeons and became known as the Buckston Browne Research Farm. Much good research was done there until it had to be closed in the mid-1980s as a result of pressure from Animal Rights activists.

In 1952 Down House was offered to and accepted by the College and became occupied by Sir Hedley Atkins, Professor of Surgery at Guy's and later President of the College from 1966 to 1969. His son, Chris, was a direct contemporary and friend of mine and I can remember spending a night with him at Down while we were still medical students. At that time the ground floor of the house was a museum dedicated to Darwin and Hedley and his wife used the upper floor as their home. He was the honorary and enthusiastic curator of the museum and many generations of surgeons enjoyed their gracious hospitality in Down House and its gardens. After his death the College hired a resident curator to look after the museum. However, during my time as President, Council decided that we were not equipped to run an increasingly important museum and soon after I demitted office it was passed first to the Natural History Museum and then finally to English Heritage, who have now developed it into a fine memorial to one of England's greatest scientists.

Before this took place we still had access to the property on which the village cricket pitch was situated and the annual match was an enjoyable social occasion. The two teams were accompanied by wives and family who provided picnic lunches, and at the end of the day there were strawberries and champagne in the museum. As President it was my duty to captain the Council team. At my school in Natal, three of my contemporaries had gone on to play for South Africa but I had never progressed further than the 3rd XI. So I approached this responsibility with some misgiving. The other problem was that one of the Porters in the College was a devastating fast bowler, which contributed to the superiority of their team. Having lost the first two annual matches rather ignominiously I decided that something had to be done to restore the primacy and dignity of Council. So I invited a number of younger surgeons, whom I had heard played good cricket, to augment our team. The result was that we won the last match comfortably and honour was almost restored, except for complaints from some of our adversaries that what I had done was not in the true spirit of the game.

My knighthood and other honours

It was customary for Presidents of the major medical Royal Colleges to be awarded an honour during or after their term of office and I was delighted to arrive home one night in November 1990 to find a letter from the Prime Minister's office offering me a KBE in the New Year's Honours list. This came earlier than I could have ever anticipated and when it was announced I was humbled by how many letters of congratulation I received. One of these was from William Waldegrave, to whom I replied:

"How very kind of you to write. The congratulations of friends and colleagues brings added pleasure. I look forward to the remaining eighteen months of my presidency with enthusiasm and pleasure in the knowledge that you are at the helm of the Health Service. You have already established a favourable impression with the leaders of the medical profession and we shall try and play a constructive role in making the new reforms work and achieving the best service for patients."

My family was also delighted. I wasn't sure how the children would react but when the invitation came from the Palace they all wanted to be present. However, this was not possible as only the spouse and two children were permitted as guests. So a ballot was held which the two younger ones, Mary and William, won. We then enjoyed a splendid occasion at the Palace, with William looking rather strange, having had his first haircut in over a year! I could not help feeling that the ceremony

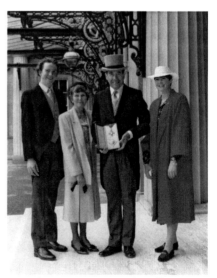

With Ann, Mary and William at
Buckingham Palace. 1991

itself was slightly unreal, as if it were more appropriate to my parents' generation than my own. Anyway, it gave much pleasure and we then went back to the Lodge for lunch with the rest of the family, including my sister Elizabeth and her husband David and my cousin Fay and her husband Richard.

Other honours came during and after my Presidency. These included Honorary Fellowships from thirteen other medical colleges, which I regarded as being earned as much by representing the Royal College of Surgeons, as by my own endeavours. There were also Honorary Doctorates of Medicine from the University of Nantes, Mahidol University in Bangkok, and much later, the University of Witwatersrand, Johannesburg. In addition I was proud to receive Doctorates of Science from the Universities of Sussex and Hull.

Fund-raising and Departure
Although throughout my time as President I gave attention and energy to fund-raising and was instrumental in starting a major appeal I cannot claim that much had been achieved by the time I left office. This was left to my successor, Norman Browse, who was very successful in getting lots of money to fund the surgical fellowship scheme that he had helped to initiate. One of the interesting fund-raising encounters I had was with Paul Getty. I knew of his interests in museums and thought he might be willing to fund refurbishment and development of the Hunterian Museum. So I invited him to lunch and gave him a tour of the Museum but nothing came from my follow-up request for money. He might, however, have felt slightly guilty about this because I then received an invitation to join his party on a day during the first test match at Lords cricket ground that summer. He had funded a whole range of boxes on the west side of the ground and kept one for his own use. This accommodated about two dozen guests and he usually had some of the great names of cricket present. Hospitality was organised by Victoria Holdsworth whom he later married and was sumptuous in the extreme. It made for a very pleasant day and I was surprised and delighted when I continued to receive similar invitations for the next two years. I suspect he may have thought I was still President of the College but did not feel it necessary to disabuse him of the fact that this was no longer so!

All good things come to an end. I presided at a Diploma Ceremony on the day before I demitted office, after which my friend Sir Magdi Yacoub delivered the Tudor Edwards Lecture.

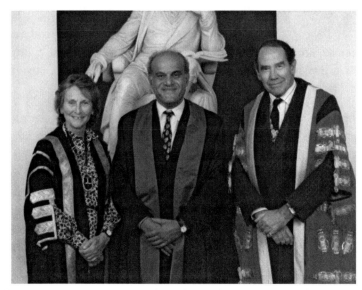

With Margaret Turner-Warwick and Magdi Yacoub – my last evening as President RCS

This was followed by a College dinner for which I had invited Margaret Turner-Warwick to be the after-dinner speaker and at which I was delighted to have all four children present. Being my last as President, I had Ann sit next to me and I closed my speech with the following remarks:

"My final and very pleasant task before I sit down is to pay tribute to the invaluable and constant support which I have had from my wife, Ann, during these past three years. I have promised not to embarrass her and I will try to adhere to that promise. For us it has been a time when, despite the hectic demands of the job, we have probably seen more of each other than at any other time of our marriage. We have enjoyed living in the Lodge enormously where, within a very short time, Ann seemed to find her own distinctive position within the family that is the College. Clearly, she enjoyed her new- found matriarchal role and will miss life at the College perhaps even more than me. Having said that I suspect we shall both look back on this as one of the happiest periods of our lives, and I simply want to thank her for her contribution to this."

Margaret Turner-Warwick gave an excellent speech and when dinner was over we had a very happy time in the Lodge with all my family and personal guests present. Next day, as the first item on the agenda after lunch, I handed over the badge of office to Norman Browse. He had arranged for Ann and his wife, Jeanne, to be present and made a generous and gracious speech in which Ann was included. Later he spoke to his "Agenda for Action" for the next three years and first impressions were most favourable. At the end of it all I felt a sense of profound relief that it was over and with much having been achieved, but also of loss that the excitement and interest of the last three years had ended.

Trekking in the Karakoram Mountains

Knowing that this might be the case, I had planned to take a three-week holiday in Northern Pakistan within a fortnight of leaving the College. This was with a small group trekking in the Karakoram Mountains in Baltistan, with the possibility of getting as far as the base camp of K2. The latter is situated on the border between China and Pakistan, and at 8688 metres is the second highest mountain in the world but more difficult to climb than Everest. Our expedition was organised by a firm in Cumbria called Karakoram Experience and we flew first to Islamabad and then to Skardu, which is situated on the banks of the Indus River and the main town in Baltistan, where we prepared for the task ahead. From there we travelled by Jeep to the village of Askole, from where the trek started. While there, one of the members of our group became seriously ill as a result of something he had eaten. I had hoped to travel 'incognito' as far as being a doctor was concerned, but I had to get involved with his treatment which involved intravenous rehydration and arranging for his return home. Thereafter my cover having been blown, I somewhat unwillingly assumed the role of group doctor.

We had about thirty porters to carry the food and equipment, accompanied by a goat that was slaughtered five days into the trip. We were responsible for putting up our own tents, mine being shared with an agreeable young man from the Midlands. Our leader was an experienced trekker and mountain climber but hopelessly disorganised over small but important matters such as remembering which food had been placed in which canister. Besides him there were seven other members of the party, mostly from very disparate backgrounds and two of whom were slightly older than me. Aileen Adams was one and the only woman in the party. She was a tough lady, having previously done arduous treks in the Himalayas and Nepal, and an excellent companion. I can remember her amusement, when asked by one of our Porters who could speak English, "Madam, why can English lady travel without husband when Pakistani lady cannot?" The other was Stuart McElvey, a retired American Army officer. Stuart was likewise fit for his age and approached the task with a dogged determination that earned the admiration of everyone.

We soon got into the routine of the day. Strong sweet tea was brought to our tent at daybreak and then after breakfast and breaking camp we would walk until noon when there would be a light lunch and a rest. We would then walk for another three or four hours before making camp for the night and having a big meal before the sun went down. The first part of the trek took us alongside the powerful Braldu River. Adjacent to some of the banks crops were grown under irrigation from the river but in other areas there were steep gorges to be negotiated involving some interesting rock climbing. The scenery became more barren as we advanced, first up the river and then on the 60km long Baltoro Glacier. The days were hot while the sun was out but it could be very cold on the glacier at night. I revelled in the splendour and remoteness of our surroundings and the simplicity of our living conditions. As we got higher, some began to experience mild symptoms of altitude sickness but the gradual nature of our ascent meant that a degree of acclimatisation was achieved. The weather remained good and we reached our final campsite at Concordia, also named "MountainThrone Room of the Gods", exhausted but exhilarated. At Concordia one is surrounded by four magnificent peaks, three of which are over 8,000 metres, and with K2 in the centre it makes an awe-inspiring sight.

Whilst there an extraordinary coincidence happened. Soon after arrival I retired to my tent for a rest and then after about half an hour who should arrive at my tent door but Ben Eiseman and Hank Bahnson, two American surgeons whom I knew well. Hank was an ex-president of the American College of Surgeons and Ben had received an Honorary Fellowship during my time on Council, after which Ann and I had visited his ranch in Colorado, where he was an avid mountain climber. They had arrived at Concordia before us and made an abortive attempt to get to the base camp of K2 that was a day's march further on. Having seen our camp they wandered over to talk to some of our party and when it transpired that they were cardiac surgeons, the individual to whom they were talking mentioned that I was part of our group which led to our meeting!

The next day we retraced our steps down the glacier and it was either then or the following day that Stuart McElvey slipped and hit his head against a sharp rock. This severed his temporal artery just above his left ear and by the time I was called back to attend to him he was covered in blood. The cut was deep and I could see his skull beneath the edges of the wound. Having controlled the bleeding by finger pressure, I then wound a long crepe bandage firmly around his head and this was kept in place for the next four days. When removed, the wound was dry and clean and simple dressings were all that were required for the next few days. Stuart remained inordinately grateful and we became good friends, keeping in touch by correspondence and a visit to his home in Sausalito when I visited San Francisco a few years later. The rest of the trek passed uneventfully and I returned home feeling much refreshed and ready for a change of life by resuming full-time surgical practice at Papworth.

Chapter 8
Master of St Catharine's College, 1993-2000

"The ease of the life of a Head of House usually leads to longevity."

John Betjeman, 1938

After three hectic years spent between London and Cambridge I returned to a more regular life style. I resumed my previous clinical duties at Papworth with the welcome agreement of my colleagues that I should remain exempt from participating in the emergency rota. I also had few administrative duties and enjoyed practising very much as I had when I first became a consultant, with most of my time devoted to seeing patients, operating and teaching. The transplant programme had progressed well under John Wallwork's guidance and was now also well served with cardiological support from Jayan Parameshwar, who had extended his role from providing a first class Out Patient service, to helping with the assessment and postoperative care of patients.

About this time I received a letter from George Duncan who had been Regional Medical Officer for East Anglia during my first fifteen years at Papworth. He enclosed a copy of an essay which he had written as part of a degree with the Open University entitled: "Cardiac Transplant Surgery at Papworth Hospital – A case study of the inter-relationships between democracy, due public process, and professional and corporate ethics." As the senior medical officer responsible for Papworth he had endured much of the political conflict, both local and at Department of Health level, that had characterised the early years of the programme, so I was touched when he ended his letter with the following words: "I hope I have done justice to the subject and the dramatis personae; for my part it was interesting and revealing to review the sources of material at an interval of some years. Above all, I remember your invariable patience, courtesy and dogged determination throughout these challenging events."

Election to the Mastership

But that was now all largely behind me, and having just turned 60 I began to reflect on what new challenges I might embark upon. However, I was in no hurry, getting much satisfaction from my life as a clinical surgeon and seeing more of my family. Then in March 1993 a new star appeared on the horizon. This was heralded by a letter from the President of St Catharine's College in Cambridge, John Shakeshaft (senior fellow), who enquired whether I would be willing to allow my name to be considered as a potential candidate for the Mastership of the College. This had arisen because the incumbent, Barry Supple, was retiring early as a result of being appointed Chief Executive of the Leverhulme Trust. The approach was wholly unexpected and although I had been elected an Honorary Fellow of the College the previous year I still knew very little about how it, or indeed the University, was run. In any event, I replied that I would like to think about it for a few days before giving him my answer.

I discussed it first with Ann who understandably was not keen to leave 19 Adams Road after having spent much of the previous three years in London. I also consulted Sir John Butterfield who was past Master of Downing College and recent Vice-Chancellor of the University. I had known him since I was a medical student at Guy's and when he came to Cambridge as Regius Professor of Physic from the Vice-Chancellorship of Nottingham he had given me much support during the early years of the transplant programme. His view was that I would be up to the job and that I would find it very interesting. Indeed he got rather enthusiastic about it. I then had a brief meeting with John Shakeshaft, who was to chair the Search Committee, during which I agreed to be considered but asked for more information about what the job involved. My next communication from him was in late April when he informed me that I was now on a shortlist of four and that the Search Committee would like to interview me on 18th May at 4 pm. Later I would dine with the Fellows, after which I should speak for about twenty minutes on how I viewed the future of the College in the 1990s and then be prepared to answer questions from Fellows. This again all came as a bit of a surprise and I had to remind him that my request for further information about the job had not been met. For this, he promised to send me a copy of the Annual Accounts and a recent report from the Senior Tutor on the academic performance of the College. Finally, I said that I would wish it be known that, if elected, I would want to continue with my surgical practice at Papworth for at least a few more years. This I thought would almost certainly count against my candidacy. However, apart from wanting to continue with surgery, I felt I owed it to the hospital and my colleagues, who had already been very understanding about the time I had spent away during the three years of my Presidency.

Ann left for a pre-planned holiday in South Africa a few days before my interview and was not due back until early June. She made it clear that she would find it difficult to leave Adams Road but generously said she would support whatever decision I came to. I had some reservations of my own. Being head of an Oxbridge college had certainly never been part of my life-plan and I could not help questioning whether I had the necessary qualities to make a success of the job. However, I decided to go ahead with the interview and the ensuing "trial by dinner". And because I thought it unlikely the Fellows would elect someone who wanted to remain in surgical practice, and because I didn't care too much if I was not chosen, I was prepared to present myself quite naturally and without any of the tensions associated with desperately wanting a job.

When the time came I was pleased to find the younger Fellows well represented on the Search Committee and the interview, which lasted one and a half hours, was friendly and constructive. Likewise my talk after dinner seemed to go well. I spoke first about my background and previous professional activities and then went on to describe what I saw as the purpose of the College; namely to attract high quality undergraduates and then to promote their academic, intellectual and social development to the full potential, whilst providing a satisfying and enjoyable environment for Fellows for their teaching and research interests. I saw the role of Master as being the head of an extended family with a whole range of ceremonial, social and administrative functions, both within the College and the University at large. I touched on some of the problems I had identified such as the current somewhat mediocre academic performance and the importance of integrating the graduate students more into the affairs of the College. And I concluded with an analysis of the financial situation and the need to increase the endowment through a more active Development Campaign. This all seemed to be well received and it was then followed by more drinks in the Upper Gallery where I was able to mix with and be questioned further by individual Fellows.

I must have been the last of the four short listed candidates to be interviewed (I never learned who the others were), because three days later I was phoned by John Shakeshaft to say that at a meeting that afternoon the Fellows had decided unanimously that they would like me to be their next Master. I was both flattered and surprised and having responded that I could not give an immediate decision I agreed to receive a delegation of four senior Fellows at my home two days later, which was a Sunday. My daughter Mary was with me at the time and she provided morning coffee for us while they, all smartly dressed, outlined more of what the job would involve. I reiterated my uncertainty as to whether I could combine it with a continuing commitment to Papworth but they did not see this as something which should exclude taking the job on, pointing out that, unlike Oxford, the head of a Cambridge college did not necessarily demand a full-time commitment and that it was not uncommon for incumbents to remain active in their previous academic or other endeavours. We left it that I would give very serious consideration to the honour I was being offered and that after discussing it further with my wife and colleagues at Papworth I would let them have my decision within eight days. I then had several phone calls with Ann in South Africa during which she reiterated her preference for remaining at Adams Road, but said she would support the move if I really wanted the job. My colleagues and the Chief Executive at Papworth were supportive and it was agreed that if I did go to St Catharine's I would continue with my existing operating sessions and out-patient clinic but be absolved from all administrative duties at the hospital. This would leave Tuesday, Thursday and the weekends for my role at the College. And so, during the next week I came to the firm conclusion that this was an opportunity not to be missed and that it would bring a whole new dimension of interest to my remaining years – a Star well worth following despite the uncertainties involved. When I phoned John Shakeshaft as promised on 1st June his evident relief was quite touching and three days later the election procedure by the Fellows was concluded. He phoned me afterwards to say how pleased everyone was with the outcome and that it had been celebrated immediately with champagne – after which I had a drink myself!

My formal induction as Master took place in the College Chapel on 27th July 1993. This was a moving experience and in the presence of forty-five Fellows I was installed the 36th Master of St Catharine's (and only the second surgeon to be elected Head of a Cambridge College, Howard Marsh having been Master of Downing from 1903 to 1915). The ceremony started promptly at 7 pm and was brief. A Latin statement from the Chaplain was followed by my Oath in Latin, which when translated read as follows:

"I, Terence English, pledge my faith that I shall rule, defend, protect and direct the College or Hall of St Catharine the Virgin, its lands and buildings, its possessions, its rents both temporal and ecclesiastical, and all rights and goods whatsoever of the aforesaid College or Hall, and I shall do all in my power to have them ruled, protected and directed by others. Again, I shall steadfastly observe all present and future statutes of the aforesaid College or Hall, with all its goods, against all its enemies. And so far as in me lies, I shall make and carry out just and appropriate corrections, chastisements, and reforms and, so far as in me lies, shall ensure that they are made and carried out by others."

I then moved from the entrance of the chapel, where the Oath had been delivered, to the Master's pew after which two brief prayers concluded the ceremony. The Fellows then lined up in seniority in the antechapel so that I could shake hands with each of them and we then all went for dinner in the Senior Common Room (SCR) for which my predecessor, Barry Supple, had kindly provided the wine. At the end of the meal I was required to make a speech, which I kept brief. After thanking them for the honour they had bestowed on me and the warmth and friendliness with which I had been received, I observed that perhaps my relative ignorance of College affairs might have some advantage because I would not be starting with any prejudices, at least none that I was aware of. I saw the need to recognise and respond to some of the pressures for change that the University sector was being subjected to but at the same time believed that it was important to preserve traditions, some of which might seem out of date but which still enriched our experience and environment. I gave the recent ceremony in Chapel as an example that could only add to and strengthen the sense of commitment I felt for the College. However, I hastened to add that I was not immediately intent on putting into practice that part of my Oath which, when translated, declared that I would make and carry out just and appropriate corrections, chastisements and reforms! Altogether, it was a delightful evening and made me feel how fortunate it was that this rather special opportunity had been granted to me.

The Role of Master
A few days later I presided over my first College Meeting. This was brief but at least gave me some idea of what to expect in future. There were

few demands during the next two summer months, which provided an opportunity to learn more about the history and current workings of the College and to prepare for my role as Master. In connection with the latter I was interested to read the following extract from Volume IV of *A History of the University of Cambridge*:

"Commonly the head of college is chairman of a group of equals, each with his own individuality to express and preserve, and the most successful have been those who could find the pulse of that strange community and draw out the best from that large pool of talent. But there is a residuum of dignity and authority in mastership too, which a man of exceptional force of character, self-confidence and adroitness in the handling of men may harness to an authoritarian regime. For those of us who have known such heads of colleges, they seem to dwell in different worlds."

I had no intention of developing an authoritarian regime, or indeed of dwelling in a different world. Within the democratic community that I perceived St Catharine's to be, I saw the role of Master to be very different from that of Chief Executive. In fact Barry Supple's parting comment had been: "You do realise Terence, that the only real power you will have is that of deciding the room allocations for Fellows!" Clearly this was said partly in jest, but I think I realised even then that the ability to influence events would not reside in the direct exercise of autocratic rule, but rather as a result of gradually gaining the confidence of Fellows in my judgement and aims. Also because of the constraints on time made by my work at Papworth, I recognised that at least for the first few years I would need to delegate to senior Fellows and College officers some of the duties I would normally have assumed. In fact this proved to be a good move, because by the time I did become more full-time I had a better grasp of some of the more difficult areas and what I should become involved in and what was best left alone.

Oxford and Cambridge are exceptionally fine universities and are unusual in their collegiate structure, with a tutorial system which results in undergraduates receiving much of their tuition as individuals or in small groups from within their colleges. Some lectures and most of the laboratory work is organised by Departments of the University, which is also the examining body. Colleges are also largely responsible for admitting their own students and herein resides part of their strength. Having a talented pool to choose from, Directors of Studies do not wish to see any of their students performing poorly and are generally supportive if a candidate they have chosen starts falling behind. Conversely most students feel a loyalty and commitment to the college that has chosen them. Another educational strength of the collegiate system is that much of the undergraduates' life comes from within their college so that they mix across a wide variety of disciplines.

It was not always thus in Cambridge. For example, when Robert Woodlark became Founder and First Master of St Catharine's in 1473 his modest institution contained no students and the few Fellows were restricted to studying philosophy and sacred theology. Woodlark was unusual in that at the time of founding 'Saynt Kateryn' he was still Provost of King's College, a position he held from 1452 to 1479. So that in Fuller's words: "Herein he stands alone, without any to accompany him, being the first and the last who was Master of an College and at the same time Founder of another." (T Fuller, "The Worthies of England, 1952 p. 446) As mentioned his college started on a small scale. However, his selection of Fellows must have been astute because of the seven who entered between 1502 and 1518, three subsequently became Masters of other Cambridge Colleges – Clare, Jesus and Pembroke.

During the 16th century students began to be admitted and in 1542 the Edwardian Statutes added "The Arts" as subjects that might be studied in addition to philosophy and theology, but it remained not legal for a Fellow of the University to study medicine until 1860. This raises the interesting point as to how John Addenbrooke graduated Doctor of Physic in 1711 despite the existing statutes, having previously qualified at the Royal College of Physicians. When he died eight years later he left about £4,500 to found the hospital that is named after him. The Master and Fellows of Catharine Hall were charged as trustees " to hire, fit-up, purchase or erect a building fit for a small physical hospital for poor people". However, owing to the dilatory behaviour of the trustees, Addenbrooke's Hospital was not opened until forty-seven years after its founder's death. Nevertheless, he would be proud to know that it is now at the heart of one of the finest academic biomedical centres in Europe.

By the time I became Master of St Catharine's the college had expanded to a Fellowship of nearly fifty, with four hundred and twenty undergraduates reading courses in all subjects offered by the University. There were also about one hundred and fifty graduate students taking a mixture of Master's and

Doctorate degrees, about half of these coming from abroad. St Catharine's has a justified reputation as a friendly and well-knit community, with good relations between students and fellows. However, recent academic performance as judged by the annual Tompkins table, in which colleges are ranked according to Final Year results, had not been good and one of the first letters I received was from an old member in which he enclosed a newspaper report of that year's Tompkins table, across which he had scrawled in red ink: "This is most depressing. Can't anything be done to improve things? An old Catsman". Our position on that occasion was 19th out of 24. Alas, when we came 2nd three years later, for which I can claim no personal credit, I was unable to inform him of this as his original letter had been anonymous.

Ann and I moved into the Lodge a few weeks before the commencement of Michaelmas term in 1993, having managed to let 19 Adams Road. The Master's Lodge, built in 1875, is a rather grand building modelled on Sawston Hall. It was built on land which was originally the site of the Anatomy School in Cambridge and which was purchased by St Catharine's some forty years earlier. This large Victorian red brick building had long been regarded by the Fellows as something of a white elephant. However, it had been extensively refurbished and modernised before my predecessor moved in and I was delighted with it. The ground floor comprised an impressive entrance Hall adjoining a large baronial style dining room, beyond which was a pleasant study. Both rooms incorporated some fine seventeenth century oak panelling taken from Old Lodge and the original buttery. There were two large drawing rooms on the first floor and sufficient bedrooms for guests as well as one each for our four children as added attractions for them to visit. The Lodge had its own private garden and was conveniently close though separate from the rest of the College. I found it ideal both for living in and for the many social occasions that became a large part of our role. These included a weekly sit-down lunch for twenty-four undergraduates that Ann and I hosted during term time. My secretary provided a random seating plan for these to ensure that they were mixed up and that new contacts were made. We also had regular dinners for our friends and members of other colleges and I would always try and have one or two of our own Fellows, plus spouses or partners at these gatherings.

My first official function as Master took place towards the end of September when I was invited to attend the Annual Dinner of the St Catharine's Society. I was seated next to the President, Bill Speake, and all went well until just before he was about to make his speech when the elderly Secretary of the Society, who was sitting in the body of the Hall and who had not long recovered from a serious stroke, collapsed. Being a doctor, I immediately went to assess the situation and was alarmed to find him unconscious and apparently pulseless. With assistance, I carried him to the adjoining SCR and having laid him on the floor was wondering what to do next as in view of his age and medical history I did not think it appropriate to embark upon cardiopulmonary resuscitation. However, I then detected a faint pulse which grew stronger with time and then one eye opened and I realised he must have just had a profound faint. So I left one of the Fellows to remain with him and suggested that an ambulance be called to take him home. Having returned to the Hall, the President gave his speech, but just as I was about to reply, I was called back to the SCR. There I encountered a burly ambulance driver who was insisting that Tom, now fully conscious, and his wife who had just arrived, be taken to hospital rather than to his home. When he saw me he greeted me by name and when I enquired where we had met he replied that he had taught my daughter Katharine Karate. Having established this degree of rapport he was prepared to follow my advice and take Tom and his wife home and I returned to give my speech, during which I was able to confirm that all had turned out well. Many of the members came up afterwards and introduced themselves to me and I went home after midnight with a warm glow that the first hurdle had been successfully negotiated.

The Fellowship

The first full Governing Body meeting that I chaired took place early in Michaelmas Term. Having read all the papers and prepared carefully for it, all went well until we came to the penultimate item on the Agenda, for which there was no paper, and which was innocently titled "Lawn on Main Court". Suddenly, however, it all became very difficult. Apparently the Fellow Gardener, a distinguished Professor of Geography, had decided to cut the lawn back over the engineering bricks, whereas before it had been allowed to extend to their edge. Unfortunately, after having done this on two sides of the Court he had stopped to assess the situation and it was then that it was noticed by some of the Fellows. At Governing Body a brisk and acrimonious debate ensued. It was claimed that traditionally the grass had always covered the bricks and eventually a motion of censure was proposed and passed by a majority vote. I was then further amazed when a second motion was proposed, "requiring the Fellow Gardener to replace the turf forthwith", which was also voted on and passed. I found the whole business quite extraordinary, if not bizarre and couldn't help wondering whether it had been put on just for my benefit. However, this was dispelled when the Professor of Geography came to see me the next morning to say that he was resigning from his position as Fellow Gardener! I remember subsequently mentioning to the Senior Tutor that I was surprised that Fellows could be so rude to each other in an open meeting, but was reassured that this was no more than a little 'static' that erupted from time to time and should not be taken too seriously.

Certainly chairing the Governing Body was a different experience from that of chairing the Council of the Royal College of Surgeons. As a very broad – and probably inaccurate generalisation - dons seemed to me to be constitutionally disputatious and inclined to want to discuss certain issues endlessly. So that in my third term I proposed that Fellows should only expect to speak once on any agenda item. This was not accepted, although I remember being congratulated by one or two other Heads of Colleges for having attempted such a bold move. In fact with time I became comfortable with the way Governing Body meetings proceeded and although occasionally tempted, I never had to remind them of Joubert's observation: "Gentlemen, the aim of argument or discussion should not be victory but progress." Contrary to my initial opinion, I also saw value in there not being an Executive Committee. Although having a large Governing Body responsible for all decisions was somewhat unwieldy, it did satisfy the democratic traditions of the College and also meant that no Fellow could complain of not being informed about what was going on. I used to meet on a weekly basis with the Bursar and less frequently with the Senior Tutor. Inevitably there were rare occasions when decisions needed to be made between meetings and then reported to the next Governing Body (GB). Usually these were accepted but occasionally knuckles would be rapped if it were felt authority was being exercised too freely.

During my time, I think there were only three occasions when I was seriously at odds with the GB. The first occurred at the beginning of the 1994 academic year when one of the new students refused on principle to wear a college gown. This was the rule for undergraduates attending formal University functions such as Matriculation and the awarding of degrees, as well as for some college activities such as Chapel, dining in Formal Hall, or any disciplinary procedure. In this case the Admissions Tutor felt that the student's principles should be respected and that she should be allowed to matriculate without a gown. I was concerned about the longer term implications of such a decision and, as a compromise could not be reached between us, determined that it was of sufficient importance to bring it to the Governing Body which was due to meet the next week. This caused considerable controversy amongst some Fellows, who argued that such a move would inevitably become public and harm the reputation of the College, make the Fellows look ridiculous and even damage the authority of my Mastership. However, I held my ground and in the event the discussion at Governing Body was controlled and informative and helped to clarify College policy in this difficult area. The final decision was that she should be allowed to matriculate without a gown, but that thereafter failure to wear a gown would exclude her from those functions where this was normally required. Indeed this is what happened and I believe she eventually graduated in absentia.

The second disagreement was more important and eventually more damaging to the College. A young and inexperienced Development Director had inexplicably been appointed in the knowledge that I was soon to take up office. She proved to be so ineffectual that we had to terminate her employment within six months. We then struggled on with a series of part-time consultants but this remained unsatisfactory and expensive. I had formed a strong Development Committee by this time but was in need of a really good Development Director to assist me and galvanise the Committee into more concerted action. Having advertised the job, we received an application from Anne Lyon whom I thought would be ideal for the job. She had just completed an excellent appeal for a local school and seemed to have the necessary energy and charm to establish good relations with our senior members and also bridge the gap in College between the Alumni office and the Development office. Because at the time I knew that there were other colleges looking for a good Development Director, I asked the Appointment Committee to consider her application before the closing date for applications had been reached. Having interviewed her the Committee agreed she was right for the job. We also agreed that although she would be placed on the appropriate University salary scale, we would need to augment this by including an element of performance related pay. In addition, she had made it clear that in order to function effectively she would need to be a Fellow of the College. As she was a Girton college graduate and had a PhD in Chemistry I felt that she had the necessary academic qualifications to justify a Fellowship and our recommendation to the Governing Body therefore included this.

I am afraid that the GB was at its most contentious when the matter came before it. We were criticised for holding the interview before the advertised closing date for applications and the concept of performance related pay was viewed with concern. Furthermore, there were grave misgivings about awarding a Fellowship to a Development Director. So although the appointment was eventually and grudgingly approved, it came without the Fellowship that both Anne and I felt was a necessary component of the job. I had the difficult task of informing her of this but did so with the promise that I would raise the matter again with the Fellowship Committee in two years time. She then took on the task with enthusiasm and within a short time had transformed the direction and momentum of the Appeal. But sadly a majority of the Fellows remained intransigent and, despite the unanimous recommendation of the Fellowship Committee that she be elected a Fellow, the best the Governing Body would do was to make her a Fellow Commoner. It was not surprising to me therefore when, soon after I left, she accepted a handsome offer with a full Fellowship from Caius College, where she was hugely appreciated and made a major contribution towards increasing their already substantial endowment.

The third problem I had with the GB related to my proposal for a possible development on one side of Main Court. A special feature of St Catharine's is the open view one has of the Main Court of the College from Trumpington Street. At the time of the Ramsden benefaction in the 17th century the plan was to close the quadrangle by building additional chambers on the East side of the Court, but money ran out and this was left open to the road which then became the main entrance to the College. My proposal had its origins in a suggestion by an old member that it would be possible to achieve the extra accommodation we needed, and yet preserve the "openness" of Main Court, if a design along the lines adopted by Peterhouse in the 17th century was followed. At that time their new Chapel was built along an East-West axis facing into Old Court with arcaded galleries connecting it to the adjoining buildings so that it was still possible to look through the arches into Old Court from Trumpington Street. The senior member, who wished to remain anonymous, generously agreed to pay for some preliminary architectural work and I engaged two Cambridge architects, Michael Walton and Jon Harris to come up with a plan.

This comprised a central building containing an auditorium with a capacity of 160 suitable for lectures, concerts, plays or recitals, and with a foyer and a basement area containing music practice rooms, piano store, dressing-rooms and cloakrooms. On the first floor there was to be a reception area and a pair of seminar rooms each accommodating 20 to 30 people. Arcaded wings would link this building with Hobsons and Woodlark on each side, preserving a degree of openness to Main Court. On the first and second floors, which extended over these wings, there would be space for a library extension, seven Fellows' sets, and an equivalent number of undergraduate rooms.

I was excited by these plans and having discussed them with the Bursar brought a proposal to the GB meeting in October 1997 for preliminary consideration, after which I suggested there should be an opportunity to discuss them in depth at a College-style Seminar with Michael Walton and Jon Harris in attendance. However, the proposal was met largely with apathy and silence apart from one Fellow stating, "over my dead body will one brick ever be laid on Front Court". So much to the disappointment of our two architects, and not least to me, it was rejected without further consideration. About this time, and in keeping with tradition, my portrait was painted. I had chosen

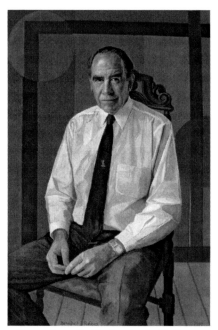

Portrait at St Catharine's College, by Benedict Rubbra.

Benedict Rubbra as the artist and between us we agreed that it should be less formal than was the usual custom. Fortunately the end product seemed to go down well with the Fellows.

On the whole during the seven years of my Mastership, relations with the Fellowship, both individually and as a corporate body, remained good. I had personal interviews with all of them during the first two terms and tried to establish an open and accessible style. I took lunch in College whenever I was free and enjoyed presiding at High Table, which was available most evenings except Saturday. In this connection, despite six years of tuition at school, my Latin had never been good and I approached the two College graces with some misgivings. I thought I was doing well enough, until towards the end of the first term the President kindly came to see me to ask if I could ensure that during the Ante Cibum grace I made a pause between "nobis" and "Domine"!

I regarded one of my most important tasks as that relating to the election of new Fellows. Unlike Oxford, where University lecturerships are tied to College Fellowships, no such arrangement exists in Cambridge. There are arguments for both but on the whole I think the procedure followed by Cambridge is better. If there is a teaching need in a particular subject, the first attempt is to try and attract a newly appointed or existing University lecturer to an appropriate College Fellowship. If this fails, then consideration is given to appointing a College lecturer with which is awarded a Fellowship. In the latter case, the full employment costs are borne by the college, as there is a more arduous teaching requirement than for a Fellow whose salary is paid by the University, who also has departmental teaching duties to fulfil. In both instances, however, the Cambridge Fellow has the knowledge that he or she has been chosen by a college, rather than having been assigned to one as is the case in Oxford, and hence might feel a greater commitment to it. I regarded that one of my responsibilities was to remain informed about where our teaching needs lay and to keep a lookout for possible additions to the Fellowship. Then, if someone seemed suitable, I would bring this to the attention of the Fellowships Committee for further consideration.

The Fellowship had expanded quite rapidly during my predecessor's Mastership and we were able to provide teaching for nearly all subjects offered by the University. There was also a good balance in age between senior and more junior Fellows. Where, however, there remained a serious imbalance was in the proportion of women Fellows, of whom there were only four when I arrived. By the time I left we had managed to increase their number to nine, and importantly, half of the eight Research Fellows were women.

This latter category of Fellows made an important contribution to college life. A Research Fellowship competition was held each year, alternating in the broad categories of "The Humanities and Arts" and "Sciences". These were tenable for three years and as well as a small but reasonable stipend, successful candidates were given room and board in College. No teaching was required of them so they could pursue their research without distraction. I did, however, make it clear that they should make an effort to join in some of the corporate activities of the College, and that in particular we hoped they would dine regularly at High Table, where the older Fellows were always interested to meet them and hear about their research. These Fellowships were originally funded entirely by the College but during my time I managed to get four of them endowed, either by industry or by generous senior members.

At the other end of the Fellowship were the Honorary Fellows. This was an honour the college gave sparingly. It included the two great contemporary knights of the theatre, Sir Peter Hall and Sir Ian McKellen and during my time only six additional Honorary Fellowships were awarded. These were Barry Supple (my predecessor); Professor Cham Tao Soon (President Nanyang University, Singapore); Sir Michael Peckham (Head of NHS Research); Jonathan Bate (Professor of English Literature, University of Liverpool); Jeremy Paxman, and the poet and playwright Francis Warner.

The Undergraduates

As Sir Peter Swinnerton-Dyer, my predecessor but one, said to me before I started: "Don't forget, the College exists largely for the benefit of the undergraduates", and in this I think St Catharine's record was a proud one. Inevitably there were occasional lapses in either performance or behaviour – or sometimes both – but on the whole they worked hard, played hard, and gained hugely from the very special benefit that an Oxbridge education can offer. This perhaps is best reflected in a piece the retiring JCR President, Jonathan Rudoe wrote in 1998:

"We will soon face the world with a small piece of paper from the Senate House denoting a degree as a tangible sign of our work, but I think we will also take away much more; friends, memories, personal achievements, learning (in the widest sense of the word) and also a small piece of the College spirit to journey with us in the future. We may never be able to put our finger on it, but we will know that our time at St Catharine's has had a lifelong impact on us, with our own particular experiences ever-present in whatever we go on to do."

I found my interaction with the undergraduates endlessly interesting. As mentioned previously, Ann and I held a weekly lunch for them in the Lodge, during which we entertained the 1st years during Michaelmas term, the 2nd years during Lent term, and the 3rd and 4th years during

Easter term. There were also special dinners in the Lodge for the Choir and the officers of the JCR, and MCR and other College societies and Clubs. I also promoted College sporting activities, both male and female, and because of the interest I showed in this I had the privilege of being elected a member of the Kittens Club. This is the College male sporting club and, at the dinner in Hall when I was admitted to membership, I had to go through the same initiation ceremony as other new members. This comprised eating a large chunk of cat food from a saucer without the use of hands. The equivalent female club, the Alley Cats, of which of course I was not a member, initiated their new members by kitting them out in their traditional dress – bin bags, ears and tails.

The Graduates
As with other colleges, graduate numbers had grown rapidly during the preceding two or three decades and now amounted to about one hundred and fifty. Approximately half of these came from countries outside the United Kingdom and some found it difficult to adjust to Cambridge. A few applicants expressed a preference for a particular college but most applied direct to the University and were then distributed randomly to colleges, although graduate tutors did have some choice if they chose to exercise this. In any event, although attached to a college, their academic activities took place entirely within university departments and it seemed to me that we were providing little for them beyond help with their accommodation and an MCR in College for their social use.

In discussion therefore with the Graduate Tutor I took steps to try and make them feel more part of the College. This comprised nominating two of our Fellows, one from Science and one from the Arts, as Mentors who would work with the Graduate Tutor and provide more help and advice when needed. We also established termly dinners in Hall when Fellows dined with graduates, after which we were usually invited back to the MCR for drinks and further conversation. Both of these initiatives were appreciated and seemed to integrate graduates more firmly into college life.

Sport
St Catharine's had at one time been a very strong sporting college and in 1934 the whole of the College rugby three-quarter line were Internationals. With the advent of Graduate Colleges in Cambridge these tended to dominate many sports and it was from them that the majority of current

rugby and rowing blues are drawn. However, the league and the College Cuppers, were always strongly contested and I had the pleasure of supporting our rugby team whenever possible.

In this regard, an interesting event happened on an occasion during a match against Jesus played on their ground. During the second half our Captain was injured and so I went on to the field to see what had happened. I found him stretched out and in great pain from what I thought must be a dislocated patella of the knee. Not being an orthopaedic surgeon I had never had to deal with this before, but decided that it was worth trying to reduce it to lesson his pain. So I told him what I was going to do and to grit his teeth while I manipulated the patella beck into position. The result was gratifying and the crowd who had gathered round, including the Captain's girlfriend, were impressed. So when the referee exclaimed with admiration: "You must have done many of those, Sir", I did not think it necessary to disabuse him. That year in the College Cuppers competition, St Catharine's defeated the first division champions and went on to a spirited performance against a blues-laden Hughes Hall side in the final. Only once in the previous twenty years had the college side reached this stage of the tournament. And the next year we had the honour of one of our undergraduates, Michael Haslett, captaining the University XV.

Soon after my election as Master I also became involved in University sport when John Butterfield asked me to become a Director of the Hawks' Club. This is the University's male elite sporting club with members being elected by a Resident Committee of top athletes. The Directors are responsible for the financial affairs of the Club, including the award of sporting bursaries and for maintaining the excellent accommodation provided by the Club House in Portugal Street. Although women were permitted as guests, their exclusion from membership of the Club had long been a source of embarrassment and irritation to the University. When I took over from John Butterfield as Chairman, the Directors tried on two separate occasions to persuade the Resident Hawks to share the accommodation with the Ospreys Club. The latter was the equivalent, though more recent, women's sporting club who at that time had no home of their own. On both occasions we failed, one of the arguments being that this would simply be the first step towards women being granted full membership of the Hawks'. However, partial resolution of the problem was achieved when Jean Gurdon, wife of the Master of Magdalene College, generously managed to provide the Ospreys with accommodation. Before leaving St

Catharine's I was able to invite both committees to a successful dinner party in the Master's Lodge. However, they still remain separate.

Music and Chapel

St Catharine's is also particularly strong in music. This stemmed from the long association of Peter le Huray with the College, who brought the St Catharine's Chapel Choir to unprecedented levels of excellence and amongst one of the best mixed choirs in Cambridge. He was also a gifted and inspirational teacher for whom generations of Organ Scholars had reason to be grateful. He had held the organ scholarship in 1948 and then, during an exceptional academic career, became Fellow of St Catharine's and University Lecturer in the Music Faculty. Alas he died the year before I became Master but music in the College continued to flourish at all levels.

Besides singing in chapel and giving concerts elsewhere in Cambridge, the choir made annual overseas tours during the summer. During my time these included the East Coast of America (twice), France, Ireland, Italy, Croatia and Slovenia. One of the most successful tours was to South Africa as a result of an invitation to sing at the Grahamstown Arts Festival. The tour got off to a great start at Plettenberg Bay, where the choir was also able to enjoy a 'braivleis' (barbecue) hosted by my brother-in-law Tom Dicey and his wife Annetjie on their farm, and other venues included East London and Cape Town.

Other musical activities at St Catharine's included Wednesday lunchtime recitals and Friday night chamber concerts, both held in chapel during full term. More formal concerts were put on by the college Music Society in the West Road Concert Hall or the University Church of Great St Mary. There were also the occasional ambitious musicals such as West Side Story, Joseph and the Amazing Technicolour Dreamcoat, and Bugsy Malone, all of which were hugely enjoyed by the undergraduates.

One of the most memorable musical events during my Mastership was a concert given in honour of Lord Menuhin's 80th birthday in 1997. He had been elected an Honorary Fellow in 1973 for a contribution he made to the 500th anniversary celebrations of the founding of the College, but had only visited the College once since then. So I was delighted when he accepted my invitation to a special concert in chapel followed by dinner in Hall. He agreed to spend the night in the Lodge and was a most charming and interesting person to have as a guest. Our top musicians gave a fine performance for him in chapel, which was packed to overflowing. The dinner afterwards was attended by Fellows of the college and members of the choir and Music Society and after toasting his health on this very auspicious occasion, he gave a most interesting speech concentrating on the musicians in the Hall, and one which I am sure they will always remember.

Another memorable concert, this time in association with the Yehudi Menuhin School Orchestra, was held during my last year. This was at St Peter's Church, Eaton Square in London and was open to the public and heralded the launch of the Chapel Organ Restoration Fund. Paul Watkins, who matriculated at St Catharine's in 1988, and who himself had attended the Yehudi Menuhin School as a pupil, had become a cellist of international standing and generously offered to particpate in the concert and conduct the orchestra. This proved an outstanding success both in the enjoyment of the two orchestras, the quality of the music and the sum of money raised.

Old Members and Fund-Raising

Having committed myself to fund-raising, it soon became apparent that in this respect the old members – as our alumni are called – were a neglected resource. I decided I wanted to be a 'visible' head of the College and that ideally the Alumni Office should be joined with the Development Office. Owing to the initial difficulties with respect to appointing a good Development Director, the latter was not achieved until late in my Mastership but during the early years I made strenuous efforts to get to know as many old members as possible. This involved holding meetings with the Regional Committees in London, the rest of England and Scotland and an early visit to the United States and Canada where I met members in New York, Detroit, San Francisco, Los Angeles, Ottawa and Toronto. In conjunction with the Development Campaign Group, which was established soon after my arrival, and which was ably chaired first by Roy Chapman and then by Sir Geoffrey Pattie, we held dinners in College for various groups of old members such as those from the City, Law, Medicine and Engineering. The plan here was to get each group competing to raise more money than the others. This worked well and also brought old members back to the College, which they clearly enjoyed and which hopefully may have an impact on future legacies. To this end we established a Woodlark Society, made up of those who committed to providing a legacy for St Catharine's and for whom we had an annual dinner.

Early on Peter Mason, an old member, encouraged me to join the Athenaeum Club in London, so that I could dine potential major benefactors in an environment conducive to asking for their support for the College. As with all fund-raising, it was impossible to predict who might or might not respond to such requests, but I believe this was also time well spent in helping members to engage more favourably with the College. Quite apart from the fund-raising aspect, I enjoyed these personal contacts and made many good friends amongst the old members. By the time of my departure the College endowment had increased from £14,166,000 to £24,200,000 and we had also achieved a major building expansion of St Chad's, after which it was able to house all of our second year undergraduates and for which the Wolfson Foundation contributed £500,000.

Besides my role at St Catharine's there were other University duties to become involved in. Alternating with the President of Queen's College, I deputised for the Vice-Chancellor in the annual degree ceremony for our respective graduates held in the Senate House. This was always followed by a delightful garden party back at St Catharine's, attended by proud parents and relieved students. I also chaired the University Health Services Committee and the Occupational Health Committee and was a member of the Committee for Honorary Degrees for two years. During 1998 I served on the University Council as one of four College representatives. I found this a somewhat depressing experience. It seemed to me that procedures were cumbersome and that the democratic process whereby a relatively small number of members acting through the Regent House could obstruct important decisions was not the best way of conducting business. The Vice-Chancellor, who chaired Council, also had to put up with one very disruptive member, who frequently created an unpleasant atmosphere. However, I came to the conclusion that although the manifestations of academic democracy in both Oxford and Cambridge could be irritating and frustrating, they were at the heart of these two great universities and reflected something that had more strengths than weaknesses.

An unusual university-related event occurred through my friendship with Christiaan Barnard who I had got to know as a result of our mutual transplant activities. This was heralded by a telephone call from South Africa in which he told me that one of his ex-father-in-laws, who was very rich, wanted to establish a cancer research centre in memory of his wife who had recently died from breast cancer. The individual in question, Frederick Zoellner, was a German who had emigrated to South Africa after the war, There he had made a large fortune and Chris had married his daughter, Barbara, when she was 19 and he 48. Zoellner later retired to Switzerland and his initial suggestion was that the research centre might be based in the Max Planck Institute in Germany. However, Chris expressed the view that it would be better placed in Cambridge and this was the reason for his phone call. I was excited by the prospect because I was aware of the fact that Cambridge had a first class clinical oncology service and that a cancer research unit would fit nicely between this and the basic science being pursued in the prestigious Laboratory for Molecular Biology. So I discussed the matter with the Vice-Chancellor who was also enthusiastic and who suggested that we should ask for £1.75 million to endow the Chair. I relayed this to Chris and there then ensued protracted negotiations during which he visited Cambridge a number of times, acting as an intermediary between Zoellner and the University. Eventually, however, the agreement was finalised and I was able to heave a sign of relief. This, however, was short lived as I then received a phone call from Chris saying that he was hard up and wanted a present for his labours. I replied that I was sure the University would want to acknowledge his help but he pointed out that he wanted 'a large present' and mentioned a substantial sum of money. Understandably, the Vice-Chancellor and the Treasurer of the University were scandalised when I told them this. However, eventually a compromise was reached whereby Chris was paid an annual retainer for continuing to act as a fund-raiser for the Chair for the next five years. He did not raise any more money and sadly Zoellner died shortly before the opening ceremony of the cancer research unit. However, the first and current holder of the Chair, Professor Ashok Venkitaroman, has proved an outstanding appointment and his department is now an important component of the Cancer Research Institute on the Addenbrooke's campus.

Chapter 9
President of the BMA; the Audit Commission and Holidays
(1993 – 2000)

Apart from the College and the University I had many other activities to keep me busy during my time at St Catharine's. Symptoms from my duodenal ulcer, though much improved while I was at the College of Surgeons, were still proving troublesome a year after my return to full duties at Papworth. So with my dual role at the hospital and St Catharine's I decided that the time had come to have something definitive done about this. My physician, Dr John Hunter, agreed that I was one of those few cases that had not responded fully to all that medical treatment could offer and referred me to David Dunn for an operation. I admired David both as a person and as a surgeon and was delighted when he said he would take me on for an appropriate procedure. This was undertaken after the end of my first term at St Catharine's and was a great success, making me wish I had insisted on having it many years earlier. Sadly, David had to undergo chemotherapy for cancer soon after he operated on me and died two years later.

I continued to enjoy operating at Papworth but could see that with the Presidency of the British Medical Association due to start in June 1995 I would not be able to cope with all three jobs. So, somewhat reluctantly, I set my retirement from Papworth and the National Health Service for the end of September that year. This proved to be a moving occasion. There were presents from the hospital and the Chief Executive had prepared a book in which he had pasted letters from colleagues, patients and politicians from throughout East Anglia and further afield, all of which were much appreciated. Of special importance to me was the attendance at my farewell celebrations of eleven of the early transplant patients, sharing one hundred and thirty-one years of life since their transplants between them

The British Medical Association.

My term as President of the BMA started, as is the custom, with the Presidential Address held towards the end of the Annual Representatives Meeting, which that year was held in Harrogate. I chose as my subject "Four Decades of Cardiac Surgery 1955-95", and was able to incorporate my experience with many of the great surgeons I had worked for such as Lord Brock, Sir Thomas Holmes-Sellors, Donald Ross, John Kirklin and Norman Shumway. I talked first about the three main components of surgery, namely craft, technology and science and then about the early years of heart surgery including the development of the heart-lung machine. The latter heralded the era of 'open heart surgery' whereby vital organs could be supplied with oxygenated blood while the heart was stopped in order to repair defects within it. I then went on to describe the huge benefits that coronary artery surgery had conferred on mankind, leading finally to my own interest in replacing those hearts that had been damaged beyond recovery.

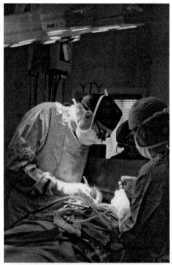

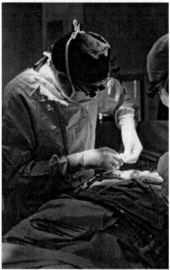

Operating at Papworth

At the end of my address, I could not help reading out the fax I had received at lunchtime from my daughter Mary, which read:

Dear Dad,

Katharine and I would like to wish you lots of luck this evening. If anyone falls asleep it will probably be because they have drunk too much port – we

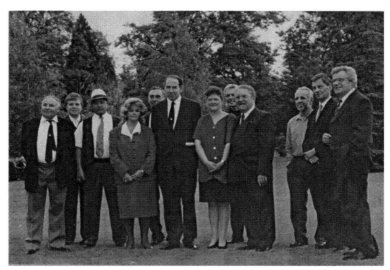

With 11 heart transplant patients celebrating a total of 131 years of life
since their operation. September 1995

know you will do well. Remember to thank your wife, children and dog for
all their love and support! Have a lovely time. With fondest love, Mary."

The BMA prides itself on being a very democratic organisation. Indeed
when Reggie Murley, who had served on its Council some years earlier,
heard that I was to become President, he responded: "Ah dear boy, the
BMA, the bloody BMA, drowning in seas of democracy". This was not my
experience and I came to respect the way it was run and, more important,
value the contribution it made not only to the medical profession, but
also to medicine in Britain generally and the NHS in particular. The
role of President is largely ceremonial, but I was assiduous in attending
Council and the main committees, where my presence seemed to be
appreciated. The Chairman of Council, Sandy Macara, and the other
chief officers of the association were helpful and friendly and provided the
necessary guidance when called for. Altogether I found it an interesting
and enjoyable experience.

A few months before I assumed office, the Secretary telephoned to apologise
that the biennial conference in October would not be able to be held
in Sri Lanka as planned, and that alternative arrangements were being
made to hold it in Cape Town. Of course I was delighted by this turn
of events and Ann and I used it to have a preliminary holiday in South
Africa. We went first to Fugitives' Drift Lodge, where I had been before

and where David Rattray used to tell the dramatic stories of the Battles of Isandhlwana and Rorke's Drift, and then on to visit relatives in Natal before going to Cape Town where we met up with the rest of the large party. The joint conference with the South African Medical Association lasted three days during which we were treated with great hospitality. In my Opening Address I was able to refer to my long links with the country, my paternal great grandparents having arrived in Cape Town in 1834 after a three-month voyage from Britain, and my grandfather having married an Afrikaner, whose family had been in the Cape since the late 17th century. I then described how I marvelled at the political changes that had taken place during the preceding few years, resulting in the peaceful election of the country's first democratically elected Government of National Unity. Also how this in turn had brought the restoration of international academic relations, of which our joint medical congress was but one manifestation. I concluded by observing that with political change comes socio-economic change, and that already one could see changes in the priorities and delivery of a health care system designed to embrace the whole of the South African nation.

At the conclusion of the conference many of our delegates stayed on to see more of the country, whereas Ann and I and a few senior officers of the Association proceeded to Mauritius for a meeting of the Commonwealth Medical Association. There we enjoyed a relaxed time and made more friends before returning to Britain and St Catharine's.

India and Ethiopia

I made two more visits abroad during my year as President, one of which was related to BMA business and the other not. The latter was a visit to India in December arranged by a new friend, Ramu Ramakrishna. I had met Ramu at a meeting of the London branch of the St Catharine's Society earlier in the year. He had graduated in law from Caius College and was living in Madras (now Chennai), and had come to our meeting as a guest of one of our alumni, who introduced him to me. Somehow the conversation turned to mangoes whereupon Ramu declared that India produced the best mangoes in the world. I said I knew a lot about mangoes and had to correct him in that undoubtedly the best ones came from Natal, of which I had personal experience. He would have none of this and four days later, while in my office at St Catharine's, I received a call from the Porter to say that an Indian gentleman had arrived and wished to see me. This proved to be Ramu who was then shown to the Lodge carrying with him a box of Indian mangoes that he wished me to sample. We did so sitting in my office, after which I was complimentary about their quality, but still insistent that Natal mangoes were better. Thus started our friendship and before leaving he had pressed on me an invitation to visit Madras and then inspect his mango estate in South India. During the ensuing months the invitations became more insistent and eventually, accompanied by our daughter Mary, Ann and I accepted his hospitality and had a most interesting time. One of the more memorable episodes was a visit to meet some of his family in Coorg. This involved an overnight train journey from Madras to Bangalore, followed by a lengthy road journey. Ramu, a confirmed bachelor, and Mary had never got on too well and one of their arguments whilst in the car was concluded by Ramu saying to Ann and me: "Very spirited young lady, you have, very spirited!" However, this didn't affect our friendship and we have continued to keep in touch over the years.

The other interesting trip, this time for the BMA, was to Ethiopia which occurred towards the end of my presidential year. The Association received many invitations to send one or more representatives to meetings of other medical organisations around the world and these used to be discussed at periodic meetings of the Chief Officers. When the invitation from the Ethiopian Medical Association arrived, no one was particularly keen to go and so I had no hesitation in volunteering. I had always considered it an interesting country and been fascinated by Wilfred Thesiger's account of his association with it, both while growing up as a boy when his father was the minister in charge of the British Legation in Ethiopia before the First World War and later, when he accompanied the Duke of Gloucester who represented King George V at the coronation of His Imperial Majesty Haile Selassie (to whom Thesiger's wonderful autobiography "The Life of my Choice" was dedicated). My other reason for volunteering was a desire to visit the Fistula Hospital in Addis Abbaba. This had been established by a husband and wife missionary team from New Zealand who soon after their arrival became aware of the terrible affliction suffered by girls who married young, became pregnant soon after puberty and then had an obstructed labour due to a disproportionately small pelvis. This often resulted days later in the passage of a macerated foetus and the development of a fistula between the vagina and/or the bladder or rectum. Catherine Hamlin and her husband Reginald set about tackling this problem and with charitable support built a hospital in Addis to deal specifically with girls suffering from the condition. I knew of their work as Catherine had been awarded a prize by the Royal College of Surgeons in recognition of their achievements. Her husband had died by then but during his life they used to operate at the same time on separate tables in a large but simple operating theatre. One of the young girls, who had been treated successfully, did not want to go back to her village and chose to remain in the hospital and helped first in the wards and then in the operating theatre. After a while the Hamlins began to use her as an assistant, initially holding a retractor and then gradually becoming involved with more complicated parts of the procedure. In this way her training progressed to the extent that she became proficient in carrying out all aspects of the operation on her own, so that when Catherine's husband died she was able to operate independently. By the time of my visit she was doing the bulk of the surgery and helping to train visiting surgeons in this difficult procedure; a truly remarkable achievement for one who had received no formal education let alone medical training. The annual meeting of the Ethiopian Medical Association went well and my attendance seemed to be appreciated. Ann and I were again shown much warm hospitality, including a short but interesting tour in the north of the country, spoilt only by one of the worst gastro-intestinal upsets I have ever endured.

As my term of office drew to a close I experienced an increasingly busy time, both generally and with BMA functions, as illustrated by the following notes:

11 June: Gave the Raven Lecture at the Royal College of Nurses: "Doctors and Nurses: an evolving relationship"

21 June: Speech at BMA conference at Sidney Sussex College

23 June: BMA Annual Meeting at Brighton

23 June: Welcome Reception Dinner and speech

24 June: Civic Reception speech at Brighton

24 June: Overseas Graduates Dinner and speech

27 June: St Catharine's Graduands Dinner and speech

28 June: Spoke at funeral of my friend Morkel Van der Merwe

2 July: Inaugural Lecture: Lewisham Academic Centre, "Medicine in the '90s – The team approach"

4 July: Address to the Graduates – Hull University

5 July: Speech at dinner for Yehudi Menuhin's 80th birthday

So ended an enjoyable and interesting year with the BMA, after which I was pleased to be able to devote more time to St Catharine's. There were, however, still other commitments I had acquired along the way that added to the overall interest of my days. Amongst these was the rather surprising role of Deputy Lieutenant of Cambridgeshire. When approached about this by the Lord Lieutenant, James Crowden, at the beginning of 1996, I indicated that I would be loath to wear uniform as I had escaped military service both in South Africa and in Britain. However, he reassured me this was not necessary and then when I asked him to tell me more about the role he responded by saying that perhaps the most arduous duty would be attending funerals of other Deputy Lieutenants! On this basis I felt comfortable to accept and indeed was proud when my appointment was recorded in the London Gazette on 10th May. This helped to enlarge my circle of acquaintances in the county and James Crowden became a firm friend.

Other activities were related to my background in medicine. I served as Chief Medical Adviser to BUPA – the British United Provident Association – from 1991-1999, and during six years at St Catharine's I was also a member of the Audit Commission. This again was a most interesting experience. Margaret Thatcher had established the Commission at the beginning of the 1980s to bring economy, efficiency and effectiveness to Local Government and subsequently the Health Service came under its regulation. It was because of the latter that I came to be appointed one of the two commissioners with a medical background; Donald Irvine a GP from Newcastle, and later to become President of the General Medical Council, being the other. The Audit Commission itself was efficiently and professionally administered and both the Chairman, David Cooksey, and the Controller (Chief Executive) Andrew Foster, were exceptionally able people. Besides being responsible for auditing public bodies such as local councils and NHS hospitals, the Commission produced authoritative reports on work related to these bodies, which auditors then used to improve economy, efficiency and effectiveness in the institutions for which they were responsible. I believe it was a grave mistake when Alan Milburn removed the NHS from the Audit Commission's remit during his term as Secretary of State for Health in Tony Blair's first Labour government.

During my last three years, I also became a non-executive Director of Papworth Hospital. This occurred only two years after my retirement so I was surprised to be asked, but apparently the Board felt they were not being kept sufficiently well informed by the then Medical Director, and that it would be desirable to have someone else on the Board who knew the hospital well. I first consulted some of the senior members of staff and as the general consensus seemed to be favourable to my joining the Board I accepted the position. This in turn gave me a comprehensive insight into the way the hospital functioned and a realisation of how well we were served by our Chief Executive, Stephen Bridge, and the Finance Director. An additional but less arduous appointment was that of Governor of the Leys School in Cambridge. The school had served my eldest son, Arthur, well and I was pleased to be able to give back something in return. The Governors' meetings, which took place on Saturday mornings, will be remembered amongst other things for the clouds of cigarette smoke which used to issue from two senior governors, Lady Trumpington and John Bradfeld, who always sat on a bench well behind the main table so that they could smoke at will and in the belief that this would not bother others.

Holidays

Throughout the seven years in the Lodge life was not entirely determined by work and I enjoyed some good holidays. I continued to take our children on an annual skiing holiday. They were all adults by now but the tradition persisted that if they came with Dad, Dad paid so they nearly always did. By this time they were all much better skiers than me but I still enjoyed the sport and loved the opportunity of being with all four of them. They were often accompanied by friends and two of the more regular and nicest ones, Rachel Harling and Jeremy Crowther, subsequently married into the family.

There were also a few great walks. In September 1993 Arthur joined me on a strenuous walk south of Toulouse in the mountainous area adjoining the border with Spain. This was organised by 'Inn Travel' so we were assured of a good meal and a comfortable bed at the end of each day. I had always enjoyed Arthur's company and the days passed quickly. He had just completed an MBA at Nottingham University and it was good to hear about this and other plans for the future. A less luxurious but equally enjoyable walk, this time with William, took place the following September along the west coast of the Outer Hebrides. He had recently returned from Vancouver Island where he had served as medical officer to a school's exploring expedition, from where he had written:

"Whilst out here I have obviously had time for reflection during which I have realised how fortunate I have been throughout life and in particular the last 7 years since leaving school. I have also realised that I may not have always expressed how grateful I am to you both for your constant love and support of which I am very well aware. So thank you both very much for being there and helping in those hundreds of different ways. I feel that I want for very little indeed. So until I see you at the end of the month I hope all continues to go well and with lots of love, William."

I was keen to receive a debriefing on his Canadian trip and as he still had some free time before taking up a three-month posting in a Trauma unit near Cape Town, I was able to persuade him to accompany me to the Hebrides. It proved to be an idyllic holiday. We travelled by overnight train to Fort William and then by ferry to Castlebay on the southern tip of Barra. From there we walked, mainly along the west coast, of the successive islands of South Uist, Benbecula, North Uist, and South Harris. We were blessed with fine days and no rain and the terrain was quite different from anything I had previously experienced. As far as accommodation was concerned, whilst staying at a B and B we would explain to our hosts roughly where we intended to be by the following evening, and then ask if they had knowledge of possible accommodation nearby. This invariably proved to be so, after which we would ask them to 'phone and reserve accommodation for us, also pointing out that we would be hungry and most appreciative of dinner. And so we progressed up the western coastline of the islands, well fed and meeting interesting locals along the way – a great holiday.

A very different environment was encountered two years later (September 1998) when I joined a small party organised by a Cambridge firm 'Wind, Sand and Stars'. This consisted of a guided trek through the mountainous region of southern Sinai. There was lots of strenuous climbing up and down mountains and we camped at night in Bedouin 'gardens'. The nights were very cold and I only felt comfortable in my sleeping bag after I was lent a woolly hat to keep my head warm. The trek finished at St Catherine's Monastery where I had an audience with the head monk, to whom I delivered a St Catharine's College flag and a piece of music composed by one of our musicians especially for the occasion. I also had the chance of seeing the Burning Bush and being shown around their magnificent library with its extraordinary collection of icons. Our tour was completed by a night climb up Mount Sinai in time to see the sunrise; it being from here that Moses descended to deliver his ten commandments and from where one has a good view of Mount St Katerina, on top of which as legend will have it, her bones were laid by angels following her martyrdom.

London to Cape Town Adventure Drive

A few weeks after my return from Sinai I embarked on a 4X4 drive from London to Cape Town. This arose as follows. The previous year a Cambridge friend of mine told me how he had joined a Classic Car rally from Peking to Paris. At the time I owned a 1964 Rolls Royce Silver Cloud III and decided that should the opportunity arise I would like to participate in a similar event. Then at the beginning of 1998 I heard that a man called John Brown, who had previously been an international rally navigator, was organising an ambitious trip for classic cars and 4X4s from London to Cape Town. I had always wanted to cross Africa by road and decided this was not to be missed. So I entered the Rolls and asked the Fellows at St Catharine's for sabbatical leave during the Michaelmas term. I thought it was perhaps better not to divulge how I intended to use the time.

I invited my brother-in-law, Tom Dicey, to join me and he responded with enthusiasm. However, as I studied the route in more detail I began to wonder about the wisdom of taking the Rolls on such a journey as it was in concourse condition. I had little doubt that it would get to Cape Town but had concerns about what its condition might be like on arrival. So perhaps my best decision, after asking Tom to be my co-driver/navigator, was to decide to do the trip in a 4X4 rather than my Rolls. In this I was fortunate in being able to acquire an eight-year old Toyota Land Cruiser that had just been driven from Johannesburg to Europe and was comprehensively fitted out for bush travel. Paul Marsh, a young South African who was selling the car for its owner then prepared it for me. He is an excellent mechanic and knew the car well, having been involved in its preparation in Johannesburg. Subsequently, I introduced Paul to John Brown, who then hired him for the trip as part of the support team.

An interesting incident happened at the Farewell Dinner before our departure from London, attended by all the family. When William left for his gap-year abroad after leaving school I had given him a £50 note in an envelope, with instructions that it was only to be used in an emergency and otherwise I would like to have it back on his return, which is what he did. During dinner I was passed an envelope from him containing a £50 note with a similar message. I was delighted!

Tom and I had a tremendous trip. It lasted eight weeks and although we were together 24 hours a day, I cannot remember the slightest lack of harmony between us. We passed first across Eastern Europe including Hungary, Romania, Bulgaria and Turkey and then through the Middle East – Syria, Jordan, the Sinai Peninsula – and into Egypt. From there we should have gone through Eritrea and Ethiopia into northern Kenya, but because of a continuing war between the two countries we had to be airlifted by two giant Russian Antonov freight-carriers into Uganda and thence to Kenya, Tanzania, Malawi, Zambia and the Victoria Falls. Whilst there two years earlier with a group from the Royal College of Surgeons en route to meetings in Zimbabwe and South Africa, I had been told by one of the surgeons as we departed that bungee jumps from the Railway Bridge were free if you were over 60 years of age. I discussed this with Tom as we progressed down Africa and decided that I should take advantage of this. So soon after arrival I went to the office next to the bridge and presented my passport to the large black man in charge with the request that I have a free jump. "No Sah", was the reply, "That finished three weeks ago". I remonstrated that perhaps as the rule had been changed so recently an exception might be made. This was followed by a big laugh and then "No Sah, I just tease you. Never been free jump for old men". I now felt rather 'boxed in' and having declared my intention to jump felt I had better go through with it. So I paid my $US90 and returned three hours later at the allotted time for the jump. Tom and a few other members of the party accompanied me, whilst I began to feel both foolish and nervous as the straps attached to the rope were tied around my ankles. I was then placed on a platform in the middle of the bridge, looking down at the turbulent waters of the Zambezi river 117 metres below as it rushed through the narrow gorge over which the bridge was built. I was told to jump with arms outstretched as if I was flying, when given the order, and after doing so can remember thinking I was going to hit one of the sides of the gorge on the way down. Instead I was arrested just above the surface of the river where

I yo-yoed a few times before coming to rest. I remained head down until an assistant was lowered on a rope alongside me and with some difficulty managed to turn me head up, after which I was hauled back to the bridge. Altogether a terrifying yet exhilarating experience but not one I have ever wished to repeat.

We then completed the journey by driving through Chobe and the Caprivi Strip into Namibia and down the West Coast of South Africa to Cape Town. There we were met by members of the family and after a great farewell dinner and prize-giving Tom and his wife Annetjie Dicey drove to their farm at Plettenberg Bay in the trusty Land Cruiser, while I followed in their car. Very sadly, Tom became ill soon after his return with a nasty lymphoma and died fifteen months later. Annetjie told me how she had prepared a book with a very full record of the trip containing lots of photographs illustrating Tom's notes from a journal he had kept, and what a comfort this had been to him during his final illness.

When we arrived in Cape Town there was a letter waiting for me from my daughter Katharine. After congratulating me on completing the trip she went on to say how she had met a new boyfriend, who lived in Swaziland and who wanted to take her on a trip through Botswana and Namibia. The problem was that he was saving up to buy a 4X4 but hadn't quite got there yet and might it be possible to lend them the Land Cruiser as it happened to be in South Africa. How could a father turn down a request like this from his beloved daughter! So after spending a few days with Tom and Annetjie at Plettenberg Bay I drove the Land Cruiser to Durban where I left it with Arthur, who had been seconded there by his Norwegian shipping firm (Gearbulk). A few months later Katharine and Michael had a great trip camping out in the remoter areas of Botswana and Namibia, sleeping either in the open or on the roof rack of the Land Cruiser if there were unfriendly animals about. After their return to Durban, Arthur kept the Land Cruiser for a while and then shipped it back to England on one of the firm's vessels. Thereafter, it took me on many other 4X4 adventure drives organised by John Brown but these will be referred to in the next chapter.

Chapter 10
Remarriage and Retirement

Towards the end of February 1998 I received an unexpected letter. This had been forwarded from Papworth and was from Judith Milne. We had first met in the autumn of 1967 soon after I started as surgical registrar at the Brompton Hospital in London. Judith was working as a senior house officer in the Cardiology Department so our paths crossed frequently and we soon fell deeply in love. However, my eldest daughter, Katharine, had been born earlier in the year and Ann was already pregnant with Arthur, so with these responsibilities I knew I had to stay with Ann and could not leave her for Judith. The disengagement was difficult and painful for both of us. Judith subsequently decided to train in Psychiatry and whilst at the Maudsley Hospital met an American fellow-trainee, Ralph Talbot, whom she married and then once they had completed their training they emigrated to Los Angeles. She wrote to me from the ship en route to New York to tell me that she was leaving England and hoped that I would find happiness in the years to come.

That was the last I heard from her until the arrival of her letter 25 years later. It was written from London and mentioned she would be coming to Cambridge for an appointment at her old college, Girton, and wondered whether I might have a few moments to catch up on what had happened to us during the intervening years. The letter took four days to reach me so that by the time I phoned she had already made her visit to Cambridge. However, I was free that afternoon and agreed to see her in London. We met at a restaurant near her hotel for two hours and then again the following morning before she returned later that day to Boston, where she had been living for the past 20 years. Before her departure I think both of us realised that our love for each other had not died and that there would be difficult decisions ahead. She and Ralph had two daughters in their twenties but their marriage had been in difficulty for some time and she was considering leaving him. My situation with Ann remained very much as it had been since the early days of our marriage. I valued her love and support and she had been a fine mother to our four children, which was particularly important during the time when they were young and I was so heavily involved with my work at Papworth. Their presence added happiness, stability and meaning to our marriage and helped greatly to make up for the lack of emotional and intellectual content that I had so earnestly hoped for. However, despite the latter, we functioned well as a family and I am sure I would never have considered leaving Ann had Judith not come back into my life.

As it was, she and I both felt compelled to see each other again after the first two brief meetings in London. I was going to Boston in May to attend a meeting of the Association of Thoracic Surgeons so we were able to meet again then. During the next year there followed a continuing correspondence and further brief meetings, both in England when she visited her brother in Sheffield, and in America when I attended another surgical meeting. By the middle of 1999 we were sure that we wanted to spend what remained of our lives together. Judith was at the time Chief of Staff of the Veterans' Administration hospital in Boston and was committed to remaining in the job for another year. Accordingly I saw no need to tell Ann about my decision until early 2000. However, during a holiday we had in South Africa in August 1999, Arthur, who was then working in Durban, joined us during our stay at Plettenberg Bay and while we were on my favourite walk around Robberg told me that one of his siblings had come across material indicating that I was proposing to leave Ann. I confirmed that this was indeed the case and it was agreed that I would arrange a meeting with Katharine, Mary and William as soon as I returned to England, but would defer speaking to Ann until after this so they could be available to support her.

A few days after my return I met the three of them in London and tried to explain the background of what had happened. Not surprisingly they found this difficult to understand, let alone accept. We all then went straight to Cambridge where I told Ann of my love for Judith and that I wanted to marry her. She was understandably devastated. The children then, and throughout the weeks, months and years that followed, were hugely supportive of her. Ann agreed that she would remain in the Master's Lodge with me until a suitable house could be found for her in London.

This was achieved two months later with the help of our friend Audrey Russell. Despite the love and attention of her children and a visit from her sister, Mary, from South Africa, Ann remained depressed and within a few months of our separation the diagnosis of early Alzheimer's disease was made. I have asked myself if I should not have recognised this earlier. In retrospect there were occasions when I was surprised she had not remembered something I had said, but at the time I simply put this down to lack of attention or absent mindedness.

Ann was against an immediate divorce so we agreed to defer this for two years when it could be accomplished in the least stressful way possible, after which Judith and I married. Initially the children remained remote and estranged and very critical of the misery I had caused their mother and for having broken up the family on which I had always placed such value. In response I could only tell them that my love for them had in no way diminished and that I hoped very much that with the passage of time I would still be able to participate in important events in their lives and regain the loving relationships we had once enjoyed. After a few difficult years

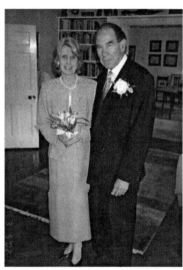

Judith and I married, 3rd May 2002

things slowly began to improve and I can now say that this has indeed been achieved. Alas, Ann's Alzheimer's progressed slowly but remorselessly. After I moved to Oxford she relocated back to Cambridge, which meant that she was closer to her friends but more difficult for the children to visit. So when it became no longer possible to manage her in Cambridge she returned to London to live in accommodation close to where Katharine and Mary were living. Inevitably there came a time when she needed more professional help and she was looked after first in a care home in Virginia Waters and then finally in St Mary's Convent and Nursing Home in Chiswick. There she received excellent care during the terminal months of her life and I was occasionally able to visit and sit with her, deeply regretting the pain and sorrow that I had caused. She died peacefully on 28th February 2009. The funeral was held in St Botolph's in Cambridge, the church she loved and had given so much to over the years. It was a memorable occasion with the church packed with family and friends from Cambridge and further afield. The address was given by the Reverend William Horbury, who knew her well, and there were moving statements from Elaine Durham, a friend and near neighbour from Adams Road, and from Katharine and William. I was most touched by the children's request that I should read the Lesson.

My decision to leave Ann for Judith was undoubtedly the most difficult I have ever been called to make. I could not help feeling then, as I still do, that this was dishonourable, particularly given the loyalty and support that Ann had given me throughout our time together. But I also know that my love for Judith was such that I could not have walked away from her a second time. During these last ten years our love has grown and strengthened to the extent that we have been able to share great happiness together. In this we are fortunate indeed and I think we can both echo Homer's sentiments when he wrote in The Odyssey: "For there's nothing fairer than when a man and a woman share their hearth together with minds that think alike".

At the beginning of February 2000, like other Heads of Oxbridge colleges, I received a letter from the Vice-Principal of St Hilda's College, Oxford, informing me that they were seeking a successor to the Principal, Miss Elizabeth Llewellyn-Smith, who was due to retire the next year. I immediately telephoned Judith in Boston, suggesting she might consider applying. Her reply was that I shouldn't get so carried away, that she had been out of the country for 25 years and that they would surely be looking for someone better known and more distinguished. Towards the end of the month she came to spend a week with me before celebrating her 60th birthday on 1st March. Two important things happened during that time. First, although we had already agreed we wanted to spend the rest of our lives together I formally proposed to her and, having been accepted, we made plans to marry in May 2002, by which time my divorce would have come through. Secondly, I managed to persuade her to see Marilyn Strathern, Principal of Girton, which had been her undergraduate college, to seek her advice as to whether she might be considered a reasonable candidate for the Principalship of St Hilda's. Marilyn, who already knew Judith from her fund-raising activities for Girton in Boston, was positive and encouraged her to apply and also offered to contact the Vice-Principal at St Hilda's on her behalf. Judith duly put in an excellent application and then, after being interviewed among a short-list of seven, she heard to her astonishment and great delight that she had been elected Principal of St Hilda's from July 2001 for a period of six years.

This made planning for our future more straightforward. Judith was able to confirm her resignation as Chief of Staff at the VA in Boston and I managed to rent a delightful house from our friends Nick and Jo Barnes from the end of September, when I was due to leave St Catharine's. This was in Harston near Cambridge and proved an ideal home for us until Judith moved into the Lodgings at St Hilda's. So at last we were settled and able to live together continuously instead of having to commute across the Atlantic for brief visits.

While on the London-Cape Town 4X4 rally, I had bought a splendid 1965 Mercedes 250SE in Botswana and had it shipped back to England. As a young man I had always wanted a white Mercedes with red leather upholstery and now at last I had one. My friend Paul Marsh gave it a complete overhaul in time for Judith and me to set off in October as participants on a London-Lisbon Classic Car Rally organised by John Brown. This was great fun and I was delighted to find that she was an excellent navigator. We spent that Christmas with Judith's daughters and friends in Boston and then at the end of January 2001 had a week in the British Virgin Islands where I had been invited to contribute to a Medical Conference organised by the Mayo Clinic. More holidays followed with a special one in South Africa in March, during which I was able to show Judith some of my favourite parts of the country as we drove from Johannesburg to the Drakensberg in Natal, then on to Zululand, the old Transkei, leading finally to the Garden route and Cape Town.

Having sold 19 Adams Road in Cambridge, I decided to stay in the property market and bought a small four- bedroom house under construction in a new estate bordering North Oxford, and a single bedroom flat in an apartment block in the centre of Oxford. The latter proved useful both as a base for Judith before she moved into the Lodgings at St Hilda's and also for me until we were married. I had planned to spend the whole of Judith's first term on a 25,000km HERO 4X4 rally around South America. This was a result of the success of the London-Cape Town rally, after which John Brown had been asked to run a similar event. It lasted eight weeks and again I was most fortunate in that two of my best friends, both still in busy cardiac surgical practices, agreed to be my co-driver/navigator. Chris McGregor joined me for the first four weeks from Rio to Lima and then Stuart Jamieson accompanied me for the rest of the trip down the length of Chile to Terra del Fuego and Ushuaia at the southernmost tip of the continent. Then back through Patagonia and Argentina to Rio from where we had started. The days were long and some of the roads appalling but the Land Cruiser, which I had shipped out for the event, performed magnificently. It was a great trip and we saw some wonderful scenery.

On return to Oxford in early December Judith had almost completed her first term at St. Hilda's. She had decided to keep a Journal of events and so we got into the habit – which has persisted – of reading this whilst drinking tea in bed in the morning. So in this way I was able to catch up with some of the more interesting and important events that had taken place while we were apart. I soon came to realise that during the next six years Judith would be heavily occupied in a challenging and demanding professional life, both within the University and as Head of St. Hilda's and that although I would be peripherally involved in some of this I would need to have tasks of my own to keep me busy.

Having left Cambridge, I thought I should resign from being a non-executive director of Papworth Hospital. I also felt that someone local should take over the Chairmanship of the Hawks' Club and I eventually managed to persuade Sir Roger Tomkys of Pembroke College to take this on. His agreement followed an amusing communication between us about two years earlier. I had noticed an announcement in The Times that a South African lawyer who had qualified at Wits University in Johannesburg had been elected the new Head of Pembroke College. During my time at St Catharine's there were two other Wits graduates who were heads of Cambridge colleges, Bob Hepple at Clare, and Dave King at Downing. So I wrote to Roger saying I was sorry to hear that he was leaving Pembroke but pleased that, as I was soon to leave St Catharine's, there would still be three heads of Cambridge colleges who were Wits graduates. To this I received a rather frosty response, indicating that he had no intention of standing down as Master and could it perhaps be Pembroke at the "other place", i.e. Oxford that I was thinking of – which of course it was!

The Hunterian Museum

There were, however, other commitments that continued when we moved to Oxford. I was able to retain links with the Royal College of Surgeons through being a Trustee of the Hunterian Museum. The Board meets four times a year and is responsible for John Hunter's great collection of specimens and art and the museum in which these are housed. Hunter can be considered the father of scientific surgery and after his death in 1793 his collection of over 16,000 dissections illustrating the comparative anatomy and pathology of animals and humans was purchased by Parliament and entrusted to the care of the Company of Surgeons, which thereupon became the Royal College of Surgeons of London. The museum, which is a centrepiece of the College, has recently been renovated and is a splendid memorial to John Hunter, currently attracting more than 40,000 visitors a year.

Northwick Park Institute for Medical Research

Another medically related responsibility I had was Chairman of Northwick Park Institute for Medical Research. This was the brainchild of Professor Colin Green who saw the opportunity for taking over the laboratories vacated by the Medical Research Council when they withdrew funding from their Clinical Research Unit at Northwick Park in 1996. Colin became Director of the Institute and managed to get Sir Stanley Peart to be Chairman of the Board of Trustees. When Stan Peart asked me to join the Board I was pleased to accept as I felt I still owed him for the difficult time he had endured as Master of the Hunterian Institute when I was President of the College of Surgeons. Then on Stan's retirement in 2001 I took over as Chairman. The Institute had some good research scientists and possessed the best large animal laboratory facilities in the south of England. However, it suffered from not being large enough to acquire major project grant funding and finances were a continuing problem. We tried to establish formal links with Imperial College but this did not get far as we soon got the impression that they wanted to "cherry pick" some of our departments but not others. Colin Green worked tirelessly both as Director and Fund Raiser and it was largely through his endeavours that the continuing success of the Institute was assured. I finally retired from the Institute in 2007 when I handed over the Chairmanship to Professor John Nicholls, who had led the St Mark's Colorectal Unit at Northwick Park Hospital. Under his guidance and a new Director since Colin Green's retirement, the Institute remains active and producing good research.

Winston Churchill Memorial Trust

One of the most interesting non-medical jobs I have had is that of Council Member of the Winston Churchill Memorial Trust. I was appointed to this in 1995 during its 30th anniversary year at which time Lady Soames, Churchill's youngest daughter, was Chairman of Council. One of Churchill's firmly expressed ideals was that British men and women from all walks of life should be enabled to benefit from travelling overseas to learn about the life and work of those from other countries. And from this experience he believed they would be in a position to make a more effective contribution to the life of Britain and of their particular community. The Trust was established on Sir Winston's death in 1965 and a national appeal was launched to fund a Travelling Fellowship scheme as a memorial to perpetuate his memory, the concept having met with his full approval before he died.

Each year 100 Fellowships are awarded by the Trust. Council selects ten to twelve broad categories within which British Citizens of all ages and from all walks of life may submit projects of their own choice. After a rigorous selection procedure Travelling Fellowships are then awarded for original and relevant projects allied to qualities of character, energy and the ability of Fellows to make best use of the opportunity made available to them. The scheme also offers the "Chance of a Lifetime" to many who would not otherwise have such an opportunity.

Council members participate in the selection of categories and also by either chairing or being a member of the interview panel responsible for a category. Somewhere between 1,000 and 2,000 applications may be received each year and the chairman of a panel may receive over 100 applications to review and reduce to a short list of perhaps 16 to 18 for interview for say 10 Fellowships to be awarded in that category. Over the years I have found it fascinating both to chair periodically the selection panel for a medical category and to participate as a panel member in one of the great varieties of other categories that are offered. These might include diverse subjects such as Science and Technology, Humane Farming Systems, Care in the Community, the Environmental, Economic and Social Implications of Sustainability, Adventure and Leadership and a host of others.

Each Fellowship is for two or three months and allows the Fellow to visit whichever countries best suit his or her purpose. The grant covers travel and living costs and on return they are required to submit a report to Council. Fellows are also presented with a silver Churchill Medallion at a ceremony usually held each year in the City of London Guildhall. It has been a great privilege to be associated with this imaginative scheme from which thousands of British men and women have now benefited, whilst at the same time adding value to their profession, institution, place of work, or community in which they live. I believe Churchill would be proud of the living memorial that the Trust has become.

Primary Trauma Care Foundation

In 1996 I was approached by Jim Ryan, who had been Professor of Military Surgery during my Presidency of the Royal College of Surgeons, to become a trustee of the Leonard Cheshire Centre for Conflict Recovery. This was in the process of being established within the Department of Surgery at University College Hospital London with Jim as Director. The purpose of the Centre was to learn from areas of conflict around the world how best to manage the period of recovery, when the fighting has stopped and most of the NGOs have gone home but when refugees and the local community are still in need of support. Our first project was in Azerbaijan and although this was planned as an academic exercise, we soon found that we were being drawn into providing aid and medical help to the refugee camps. Also, that local expectations exceeded our capacity to deliver such aid and our exit strategy was slow and painful. There followed several other similar projects but the main benefit for me was my association and subsequent friendship with John Beavis who was Honorary Lecturer at the Centre. John is a retired orthopaedic surgeon who suffered a severe heart attack in his mid-50s. After successful coronary bypass surgery he returned to work but a few months later had a bad attack of angina – chest pain – that led to his retirement from the NHS on medical grounds. However, he did not allow this to compromise his energetic and adventurous nature and he initially provided invaluable help to the surgeons of Sarajevo during the prolonged and devastating siege of that city. Then through a chance meeting with businessman Simon Oliver he established his own charity, IDEALS, International Disaster and Emergency Aid with Long Term Support, of which I later became a trustee.

Sometime during 2002 John mentioned that he would like to bring better trauma care to the North West Frontier Province of Pakistan, where there were many injuries as a result of gunshot wounds, traffic accidents, and personnel mines left by the Russians in the tribal areas along the border between Pakistan and Afghanistan. I told him of my friendship with Mohammad Kabir, ex-Professor of Surgery at the Khyber Medical College in Peshawar, who had recently established his own medical school in that city, and offered to accompany him on an assessment to determine whether such a project was feasible. We made this visit in March 2003 and were met with great kindness and helpfulness by Kabir and his family with whom we stayed. He was able to provide introductions to the Governor of the Province, who has direct responsibility for the tribal areas, and to the

Secretary for Health whose permission we needed to establish courses in trauma care in Peshawar.

Having established the feasibility of the project, John and I thought we should take the Advanced Trauma Life Support (ATLS) course. This is an American-designed course that was developed in the 1980s, and then franchised to many other countries, including Britain. So we signed up for a course at University College Hospital during which I found it interesting to reflect on who found the experience more stressful, us at the possibility of failing the exam, or the faculty at the thought of failing a retired consultant orthopaedic surgeon and the Past President of the Royal College of Surgeons! Thankfully we both passed, but having done so realised that the course was too technical and relied too heavily on sophisticated equipment and investigations for application to a developing country like Pakistan. Fortunately I then heard about Primary Trauma Care (PTC), which had been developed by a South African, Douglas Wilkinson, who is a consultant anaesthetist and intensive care specialist in Oxford. Douglas had decided to retain the principles of the ATLS course but to adapt it for use in developing countries that might not have access to the tools and equipment needed for running ATLS. The PTC course also has the advantage of being more flexible and adaptable to local circumstances and being very much cheaper. Douglas and his team had already taken the course to many countries including Africa, South America and Indonesia, and to John and me it seemed entirely appropriate for Pakistan.

So in March 2004 we took the first PTC course to Peshawar. Amongst the team of instructors were two experienced senior doctors familiar with both ATLS and PTC, two Pakistani surgeons from Peshawar currently training in Britain, and two women for whom Mrs Kabir prepared clothing suitable for the local environment. Kabir had himself been responsible for selecting the right balance of influential and appropriate members for the first course from the four medical schools in Peshawar. Some of these then went on to take the instructors' course after which, with assistance from our team, they held courses in their own hospitals. So that by the time we left nearly 100 doctors had been trained how to deal with severely injured patients. As in other countries, we found that local doctors often had the necessary knowledge but lacked a rigorous system to apply this in a way that could save life and which PTC provided.

Our first effort in Peshawar was supported financially by IDEALS and, as happens in Pakistan, word soon got around about the benefits of the course. So John was invited by the army to take a course to Rawalpindi and then towards the end of the year we were invited to Karachi. In each centre a local committee was set up to train instructors and hold courses so that by now over 2,000 doctors have been trained in PTC in Pakistan. We were also delighted when a group of instructors from Sindh were invited to hold an inaugural course in Delhi, a rare example of collaboration between doctors in India and Pakistan. Because of my involvement, Douglas asked me to become Patron of the Primary Trauma Care Foundation which is a position I have been proud to hold since 2006.

John Beavis came up with a similar proposal at the beginning of 2008 when he suggested we should consider establishing PTC courses in Gaza. Douglas agreed and so we began to explore the possibility with Medical Aid for Palestinians (MAP). Their Head Office is in London with additional offices in Ramallah in the West Bank and in Gaza. They were keen to devote more aid to Gaza so our proposal was met with enthusiasm. They wanted us to proceed directly with delivering courses but John and I both felt that, as with Pakistan, a preliminary assessment was advisable so that we could meet with local doctors and determine their willingness to proceed with such a scheme, and also to assess whether the infrastructure was sufficient to support the courses we envisaged. Initially our visit was delayed because of security concerns and then at the end of 2008 Israel launched the invasion of Gaza during which many hospitals, public and private buildings, schools and mosques were destroyed. During the three weeks of the onslaught more than 1,400 Palestinians were killed, many of who were women and children and over 5,000 casualties swamped the available medical services. There were thirteen Israeli deaths.

Our assessment visit finally took place at the beginning of August 2009. Because of our Pakistani visas John and I had to get new passports with permits to enter Gaza eventually forthcoming from the Israeli Defence Force. We went under the auspices of Medical Aid for Palestinians (MAP), spending the first night in Jerusalem before entering Gaza via the Erez crossing. Our departure from East Jerusalem coincided with a demonstration against the Israeli Eviction Police who had that morning at 6 am evicted two Palestinian families from the homes they had lived in for the previous 30 years. All their furniture had been thrown out on the pavement and two hours later Israeli settler families had moved into the houses. We were appalled by what we saw but subsequent experience confirmed that this was but one example of the policies of the Israeli

217

government towards the Palestinians and particularly with respect to what was happening in East Jerusalem.

During our week-long visit we were well looked after by staff from the local MAP office who arranged for us to meet doctors and other health practitioners from the Ministry of Health and NGO hospitals from different parts of Gaza. Generally we were met with enthusiasm for the project and were fortunate to gain the collaboration of Dr Nasser abu Shabaan, who generously offered to hold the first courses at Shifa Hospital in Gaza City. I had been given several contacts by my friend Sir Iain Chalmers, who had worked in Gaza many years before and we were impressed by the dignity and fortitude of all those whom we met. It was not difficult therefore to recommend that we proceed with two PTC courses followed by an Instructors course, with selection for the courses based on those we had met, with additional help from Dr Nasser and the Dean of the Medical School of the Islamic University in Gaza.

During the ensuing weeks Douglas and John managed to persuade James de Courcy to lead the team to Gaza and this took place in mid-November. Other members were Jeanne Frossard and Sheena Tranter, both dynamic and experienced instructors, and Graeme Groom, a friend of John's and a consultant orthopaedic surgeon at King's College Hospital, London. Again, we were well looked after by MAP and the first two courses went extremely well. Candidates for the first course tended to be more senior, with a good selection of junior doctors and senior nurses on the second course. There were twenty-four on each and from these twenty-eight signed up for the Instructors course. Before leaving, I managed to persuade Dr Nasser to be chairman of a local committee responsible for propagating PTC courses throughout Gaza, and John kindly agreed to act as external examiner for the first of these. Past experience has shown that it is helpful for experienced instructors to join the local teams for the first few courses but thereafter they become their responsibility. All of us could not help feeling great sympathy for what the Gazans continue to endure as a result of the blockade imposed by Israel. This affects every aspect of life, including health and we heard many sad stories of families being separated for years as a result of members living outside Gaza being denied re-entry by the Israeli authorities. So our gesture of support was greatly appreciated and in retrospect I couldn't help thinking that the "diplomatic" impact of our visit may have been almost as important as the medical component.

Walks and 4X4 Drives

Apart from these professional activities, I also continued to enjoy long walks and rough 4X4 drives around some of the more remote parts of the world. I had always wanted to climb Mt. Kilimanjaro, the highest mountain in Africa, and as my 70th birthday approached I decided it was then or never. So I persuaded my daughter Mary to accompany me and we joined a group of five from South Africa, meeting up with them at Moshe, the village from which most expeditions start. We had two nights there and then drove to Machama village from where the trek proper started. The skies were heavily overcast and it rained all morning as we proceeded up the trail, made very muddy by the large number of climbers on the mountain. The next day the route became much steeper but the sky was clear and we had great views both of the forest we had left behind and of Mount Mweru to the West and Kilimanjaro ahead.

The leader of our small group was a powerful but rather monosyllabic young man from Durban, but our local guide, Felix, was excellent, this being his 96th ascent of the mountain. We each had our own small tent and the food, though basic, was plentiful, supplemented by lots of hot tea. The nights were cold and we were in bed early and rose early. The days became more arduous as we progressed higher and I began to tire more easily. We arrived in mid-afternoon at the last camp before the final ascent and had a rest and a meal before embarking at 11pm for the climb to the summit. It was estimated this would take about six hours to the crater rim and then an easier hour's walk to Uhuru Peak, from where the sunrise would be observed. Alas, after four hours I was exhausted and simply could not put one foot in front of another so much to my disappointment I had to turn back in the company of one of the porters. Mary was distressed to see me go and she soon began to suffer from nausea, headache and vomiting. She was able to reach Stella's Point on the crater rim but could go no further and had to follow me down to our camp, where she collapsed into her tent. The other five all reached the summit but our leader suffered severe mountain sickness and was breathless for the next two days. Failure to get to the top was a huge disappointment for both Mary and me. But we agreed it had been a tremendous experience and I was very proud of the way she had remained cheerful and helpful at all times, despite a nasty injury to her thumb on the second day. I was even more proud when, on the final night of celebrations back at the hotel, she was awarded a special prize for "Having the prettiest smile on the Mountain"!

Mary then returned to Amsterdam where she was working and I moved on to Tsavo East National Park in Kenya where I had arranged a walking safari with a man Patrick Reynolds of whom I had heard good reports. I had decided that this would be a good move after the climb on Kilimanjaro and so it proved. Patrick ran an efficient and luxurious camp and apart from two days during the week when there was one other couple present, I was his only client. There was a lot of game about and he and his tracker always carried a rifle as a precautionary measure. He was very knowledgeable and an excellent guide and it was a delight to walk through the bush with him, while we watched many small animals and birds without the noise and smell of a vehicle. I particularly liked the early morning walks when we set off before sunrise and returned two hours later to a big breakfast. Our main camp was on the banks of a large river in which hippos cavorted, and towards the end of the week we spent two days at a fly-camp looking for the bigger game. It was altogether a delightful experience and a good way of getting over the disappointment of not getting to the top of Kilimanjaro.

Other walks followed. The next year, 2003, I joined my friend Arthur Jenkins in Tuscany. He was a professional historian who had retired to Italy where he augmented his income by taking rich Americans on walking holidays. We had known each other since South African days and I seized the chance when he offered to take me first on a walk along the Cinque Terra and then around Elba, which he wanted to survey as a potential site for one of his walks. This took place in September and it was a wonderful time to be first in Tuscany and then Elba and with someone who had such great zest for life. The following year I had little hesitation in accepting his invitation to join a walk he planned along the northern part of Sicily. This started near Palermo and proceeded through Segesta, Cefalu and the Madonie mountains to finish at Taormina. Besides Arthur and his wife Rosemary, who followed in a minibus with our luggage and picnic lunch for the day, there were five other walkers, all of whom proved interesting companions. These included Rosemary's sister Kate and her husband Ralph, Deborah Lavin a South African historian, and two American women Anne Dodge and Lyn Shields. All had walked with Arthur before and we enjoyed his capacity for interesting comment and instruction as we passed through Doric temples, Roman amphitheatres, and other ancient sites along the way. Picnic lunches were accompanied by readings from some of his favourite Italian authors. It was a special time for all of us and sadly marked the last of Arthur's walks as he died from cancer eighteen months later.

In May 2005, Katharine, baby Fred and I accompanied Mary to Lanzarotte where she was to participate in one of the toughest Ironman Triathalons in the world. This starts at sunrise with a 3.8km swim in the ocean, followed by a 180km cycle ride through the mountains of the island, and then finishes off with a full marathon of 46km. There were over 800 entrants of whom about 60 were women and we were there to support her. Mary is a strong swimmer and cyclist but not a natural runner. However, all the arduous training paid off and she completed the event in a very respectable time with Katharine and I cheering her along the way at intervals. I was hugely proud of her.

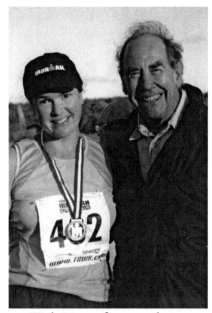

With Mary after completing Ironman Triathalon – Lanzarotte

The last of my strenuous treks was in Nepal in November 2005. This took place over nine days and was well organised by Kerr-Downey. It started with a day's sight seeing in Kathmandu during which I visited some of the magnificent Buddhist temples and palaces in the old cities of Bhaktapur and Patan. I also watched students learning how to paint Thankas, which are religious paintings found in the temples and homes of people living in Nepal and Tibet. I was impressed by the vivid colours and delicacy of the art and eventually bought a rare form of gold-painted Thanka depicting the life history of Buddha. Towards the end of the day I visited the "House of Hope", an orphanage established and funded by my surgical friend Terry Lewis and his wife Jill, and which is now a thriving community.

Then it was a flight to Pokhara by the delightfully named 'Buddha Air', during which there were glorious views of the Himalayas as we flew westward. On arrival I was met by my guide, Prem, who during the ensuing days proved an excellent companion. He had spent 22 years in the British Army, ending up as sergeant major in a Gurkha regiment, so everything went like clockwork. During the next week we tackled a number of steep trails in the Anapurna range spending nights at comfortable Lodges along the way. The day would start with a cup of hot tea while watching the sun

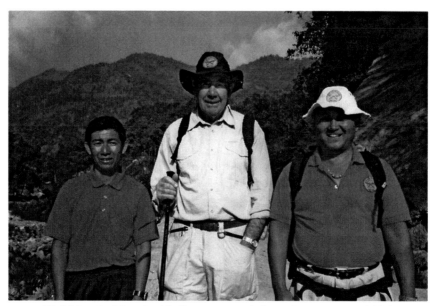
Trekking in Nepal with Prem on my left, and our porter. 2005

rise on the surrounding snow-capped mountains. Then a big breakfast, usually taken on a terrace in front of the Lodge before setting off on the day's climb. These were steeper and more arduous than I had anticipated but with rests along the way and a young porter to help with our gear, I soon got into the routine and marvelled at the changing scenery. We passed through small villages clinging to the mountainsides where we were invariably met with smiles and friendliness. The villages were often surrounded by extensive terracing on which the crops were grown. It was harvest time and everyone seemed to be busy and unlike Africa there was no begging by the children. Prem explained that this had been achieved by dissuading trekkers from giving sweets or presents to the children but instead making a small donation to the local school if they felt thus inclined. In the remoter parts we passed waterfalls, negotiated primitive suspension bridges and walked through indigenous forests thick with giant rhododendrons and wild orchids. The weather remained good, the days passed quickly and I was sad when the time came to return to Pokhara. Before saying goodbye Prem showed me round the interesting Gurkha museum and then it was back to Kathmandu and from thence home.

I have already referred to the long road trip from London to Cape Town that I did with Tom Dicey at the end of 1998 and how this was followed two years later by another 4X4 rally around South America. I had always enjoyed both driving and visiting distant parts of the world and during the next decade the adventure drives organised by John Brown allowed me to indulge in both of these activities in a way that gave much pleasure.

In his youth John Brown had been an international rally navigator and he founded his company HERO, the "Historic Endurance Rallying Organisation", for the Cape Town trip. Initially he planned participation from both classic cars and 4X4s but after the South American debacle, when many classic cars came to grief on the rough terrain, he confined further trips to 4X4s. He held them at one to two yearly intervals and his formula was to choose an interesting destination and then spend several months surveying the proposed route, seeking out challenging roads and attractive scenery, whilst arranging accommodation at appropriate intervals. Initially, modest hotels were interspersed with camping but as the years went by and his participants became older and more affluent the hotels became posher and the camp sites fewer. Also, instead of covering vast distances over eight weeks, the trips were usually confined to four or five weeks with occasional rest days at interesting places along the way.

One of the essentials for a successful trip, apart from a reliable vehicle, is a congenial companion and in this I was always most fortunate. I believed that it was best for the navigating and driving to be shared equally as in this way both would get most out of the event. For navigating we were provided with a Road Book prepared by John Brown during his route survey, which gave cumulative and interval distances between recognisable points along the way. These were then correlated with a tripmeter mounted on the dashboard of the vehicle that the navigator was responsible for operating. This was an invaluable piece of equipment, particularly when passing through foreign cities when it was impossible to decipher street names and when changes in direction might occur at short intervals. Inevitably one sometimes ended up off course and got horribly lost, but the motto in our car was "Mistakes will happen" and one then simply had to set about the sometimes difficult task of getting back on route. In later years some participants would also bring along a GPS but I found it more fun to rely on the Road Book and tripmeter.

Between 1998 and 2009 I participated in all of the events organised by HERO. After South America, Paul Marsh and I set off on "The Arctic Winter Trial" in March 2003. This was a drive from Gothenburg in Sweden through Norway to the North Cape, returning via Finland to

Helsinki, and is remembered for an accident on the third day when we skidded on a patch of black ice and ended up off the road and upside down. Fortunately neither of us was hurt and, although the roof was squashed and the windows blown out on the passenger side, the Land Cruiser was mechanically sound and we were able to continue. This, however, meant a very cold ride until we fortunately came across a Pilkington Glass factory in northern Norway where we were able to have sheets of Perspex fitted in the vacant windows.

The Arctic Winter Trial was followed by the "Grand Tour of China" in May 2004, when I was accompanied by Mary for the first half from Beijing to Lhasa and then by my brother-in-law Peter Milne from Lhasa to Hong Kong. Of the many extraordinary sights on this trip, one of the most remarkable was that of two pilgrims on a remote part of the Tibetan plateau walking the 1,500km from Golmud to Lhasa, and dropping down on their knees to pray after every third step. Apparently such a journey forms part of the path to eternal salvation. "The African Adventure" followed in August/September 2005. This proved the ideal opportunity for me to show my friend Chris McGregor some of the wilder parts of Southern Africa as we travelled through the Eastern Cape, Lesotho, Botswana and Namibia. We had stayed with Audrey Russell in Cape Town prior to setting off and she became so enthusiastic about the route that we managed to incorporate her in the second half of the trip from the Victoria Falls back to Cape Town. Next came "The Aventura Panamericana" in November 2006 when we drove from San Diego through Mexico and other Central American countries to Panama. I was again accompanied by Audrey Russell, this time with John Beavis for the first half to Mexico City and then Mary for the remainder of the trip. An amusing incident occurred while John was with us when two elderly American men, who had to leave the rally after their ancient GMC truck broke down, were heard to observe before departure that they were interested to see that "Lord and Lady English" had brought their butler with them. Thereafter John became known as "Beeves".

The "Grand Tour of India" took place in October 2007. This started from Mumbai and before setting off we were given an interesting lecture about India by a learned Sikh. He concluded by saying: "Now remember, Gentlemen, there are three essentials when driving in India; good horn, good brakes and good luck!" I found we needed all three, particularly the last. On this occasion my South African cousin, Stewart Lund, came for the first half to Shimla and then Billy Dicey, who just happened to be wandering around North India, joined me from Shimla to Goa. This was because John Beavis, who was meant to join the rally in Shimla, was unwell and only caught up with us for the last stretch from Hyderabad back to Mumbai. Finally, my cousin-in-law David Dicey, Billy's father, accompanied me on the "Singapore-Macau" rally in February/March 2008. This took us through Malaysia, Thailand, Cambodia and Laos, when I had to return to England leaving David to continue to Hong Kong.

Altogether the total distance covered on these trips with HERO amounted to approximately 64,000 miles. This was accomplished in my two Toyota Land Cruisers which, despite their age, were both wonderfully reliable vehicles. They must have covered almost the same distance by sea as on land as I used to ship them to whatever part of the world the rally was taking place in. Apart from the scenery and the driving, many good friendships were made during these events. We always travelled separately from the rest of the group during the day, usually stopping off route for morning tea and a leisurely picnic lunch. But we would meet up with the others in the evening and enjoy the companionship of our fellow travellers.

During these years the only non-HERO long distance 4X4 drive I did was through Tunisia, Libya and Egypt. This took place in November 2008 and was planned by a Belgian couple, Antoine and Maria de Hullu, who I had become friendly with through HERO. They originally planned the trip for six vehicles but shortly before we were due to leave we learned of serious security concerns in southern Libya adjacent to the Algerian border. This caused two couples to withdraw and also meant that I was unwilling to expose Mary to potential risk, as she was due to do the Libyan and Egyptian sections with us. John Beavis therefore accompanied me through Tunisia and I then did the rest of the trip on my own.

We modified our route slightly and experienced no security concerns in southern Libya, where we spent several exciting days camping in the desert and learning to drive the big sand dunes. It was here one morning while we were having breakfast that Maria, in a fit of madness, jumped into their Land Rover and drove very fast at a large dune near where we were camped. We had been talking about the need for momentum but she went so fast that she cleared the crest of the dune by at least four feet and remained airborne on the other side for another fifty feet before landing hard and smashing the suspension. Fortunately she was unhurt but the Land Rover had to be trucked back to Tripoli for repair, after which Antoine caught up with us at the Egyptian border. From there we drove far south to the interesting village of Shali which until recently was very isolated. It is situated along an extensive oasis and because of its isolation had developed its own culture and language. Then finally back to Cairo and Alexandria where I marvelled again at the magnificent new Bibliotheca Alexandrina before returning home.

While I was embarking on these somewhat frivolous but very enjoyable activities, Judith was deeply engaged in her work at St Hilda's. The major issue she had to deal with during her six years as Principal was the vexed question of whether or not the College should become co-educational. This had been debated and voted on several times before she took over and indeed she had been asked for her views on the subject when she was interviewed for the job. To this she sensibly replied that she did not feel sufficiently well informed to know what was best for the College but that she would regard one of her important roles as helping the Fellowship come to the right decision.

She was not long in the job before there was pressure from those who sought change to request another vote on the issue. This took place in March of her second year and narrowly missed the two-thirds majority required for a change of statutes. Judith was dismayed when a second vote was demanded only six months later and this too was lost by a similar margin. This meant she had the difficult task of presiding over a divided Fellowship, with firmly entrenched views on each side. However, she wisely persuaded the Governing Body to embark on a strategic review of all relevant factors before proceeding to another vote. This provided the opportunity for a thorough examination of the important financial and academic issues associated with remaining single-sex or going co-educational. At the same time the matter was able to be discussed more freely by alumnae and current students, both of which groups came to accept the need for change. So when the third vote was held in Judith's penultimate year there was a general sense of relief when this was successful. The change of Statutes was set in motion before her departure and the first two male tutorial Fellows were appointed. The Governing Body chose to defer admission of the first male students for two years so that most of the young women who had joined the College as a single-sex institution would have left by the time it became co-educational. Judith's success in guiding St Hilda's through this difficult period was a fine achievement and widely admired by her colleagues in Oxford.

Besides the College she had other University-related responsibilities to keep her busy. She chaired three Universities committees and in addition to attending the Conference of Colleges meetings, she met regularly with small groups including the Women Heads of House, the Science Heads of House and the Heads of former Women's Colleges. She was also appointed to the Academic Advisory Committee of the Centre for Islamic Studies. One of the controversies within the University that took place during her time was the Vice-Chancellor's attempt to introduce new governance procedures. This was resisted by a majority of the University dons who claimed this would inhibit the democratic processes so beloved by them. Judith was one of a group of Heads of Colleges who supported John Hood in his attempt to bring the University more in line with currently accepted practice. Although this was to no avail, his Vice-Chancellorship was successful in other respects, particularly with regard to putting it on a more secure financial basis and enhancing the efficiency of its management structures.

I kept rather on the periphery of St Hilda's although I enjoyed the social occasions and co-hosting dinner parties in the Lodgings with Judith. One of my more unexpected roles was that of a "House Spouse". This comprised a group of spouses and partners of the Heads of the colleges in Oxford. We met for lunch once a term, rotating around the various colleges, and although the male component was heavily outnumbered I always found it an agreeable occasion, as well as being a useful source of gossip about what was happening elsewhere in the University. Also, in December 2002, I was elected an Honorary Fellow of Worcester College, this being St Catharine's sister college in Oxford. I rarely dine more than once or twice a term but have come to value the association and the interesting contacts that I have made through it.

Another rather exclusive 'club' that I was invited to join soon after our arrival in Oxford was Roger Bannister's Walking Group, which he was in the process of forming. This started with nine members and during the ensuing years three more have been added as age has taken its toll. Our walks take place on the second Wednesday of each month and are planned in rotation by a member of the group. The routine is that we meet at about 10am in the car park of a pub that has been previously vetted for good food, and then walk for several hours before returning for lunch. During the years of its existence we have had much pleasure in exploring large tracts of Oxfordshire, Gloucestershire and the Chilterns and it has also proved a source of good friendship.

As Judith's term as Principal of St Hilda's approached its end in July 2007 we began to seek alternative housing in Oxford. We looked first in North Oxford and then I came by chance to view 28 Tree Lane in Iffley Village. We thought this would suit us and liked the combination of village atmosphere and easy access to central Oxford. So we duly went ahead with the purchase and then made a number of improvements before moving in. I enjoy the relative seclusion and quietness and when feeling energetic there is an attractive walk through the village and then along the towpath from Iffley Lock to Oxford. We also have the advantage of a pleasant pub that serves good food at the bottom of the Lane. Members of the village, many of whom are retired academics, were welcoming and friendly and Judith soon found herself Chairman of the "Friends of Iffley Village". Altogether, we feel comfortable in our home and fortunate to be where we are.

As already referred to, the first few years after my separation from Ann made relationships with my children very difficult. However, with time, patience and persistence I gradually won back their love and affection and now feel that we are as close as we have ever been. In addition, I have had the opportunity of getting to know and to value my relationship with my two stepdaughters, Clare and Virginia. Finally, during my retirement years, I have had the great pleasure of seeing three of my own children marry very nice people and then quickly provide me with eight grandchildren. Watching the next generation grow up and engaging with them is an endless source of fascination and I consider myself most blessed to have both a loving wife and such a fine family. And so, in conclusion, I can echo the sentiments expressed in Psalm 127, which provided the motto for Great Uncle Fred's signet ring which I have worn all these years, namely "Nisi Dominus Frustra" and which contains the lines:

"Lo, children are an heritage and gift that cometh of the Lord.

Like as arrows in the hand of the great,

Even so are the young children.

Happy is the man that hath his quiver full of them".

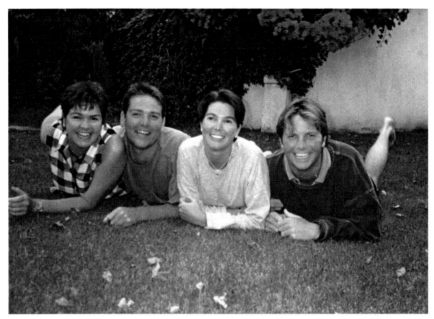

Mary Arthur Katharine William, circa 1997

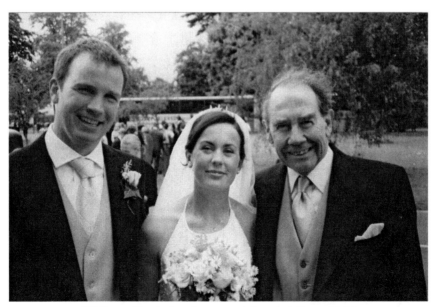

William, Rachel and me, wedding 8th June 2002

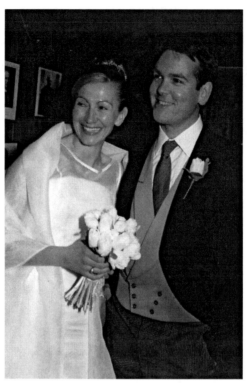

Arthur and Juliet, 22nd February 2003

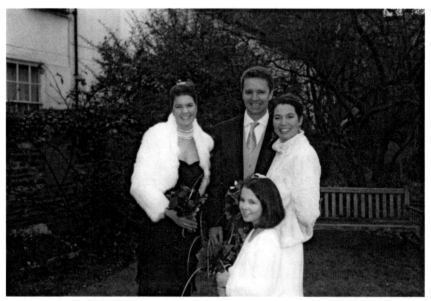

Jez and Katharine (on his left) with Mary and Lucy Shann
18th December 2004

APPENDIX

A collection of short pieces that have stimulated me over the years

Of Life and Character

"Every man is the architect of his own fortune." Old English Proverb

"All deep and earnest thinking is but the intrepid effort of the soul to keep the open independence of her sea." Herman Melville (1819-1891)

"Oh my soul, do not aspire to immortal life, but exhaust the limits of the possible." Pindar (522-443 BC)

"If there is a soul, it is a mistake to think that it is given to us fully made. It makes itself here, throughout our life, and life is nothing but this long and agonizing labour of giving it birth." Albert Camus (1913-1960)

"Obsession with the harvest and indifference to history are the two extremities of my brow." René Char (1907-1988)

"Let us judge ourselves sincerely, let us not vainly content ourselves with the common futility of our lives." William Law (1686-1761)

"The intellect of Man is forced to choose Perfection of the Life or of the Work" W.B. Yeats (1865-1939)

"Our life is what our thoughts make of it", and "There is no misfortune, but to bear it nobly is good fortune." Marcus Aurelius (121-180)

"Just as character is undone by every little fault of sloth, so intellect deteriorates after every surrender to folly: unless we consciously resist, the nonsense does not pass us by but into us." Jacques Barzun (1907-2008): "The House of Intellect"

"If I judge that a thing is true, I must preserve it."   Albert   Camus (1913-1960)

"Though Love recoil, and Reason chafe, There came a voice without reply, T'is man's perdition to be safe when for the Truth he ought to die." Ralph Waldo Emerson (1803-1882)

"Nothing is at last sacred but the integrity of your own mind."   Anon

"Does he lack organ or medium to impart his truths? He can still fall back on the elemental force of living them. This is a total act. Thinking is a partial act."   Ralph Waldo Emerson (1803-1882): "The American Scholar"

"If I had wanted to throw off all forms of constraint, it would have been in my power to cause my complete ruin and that of everyone around me. The first thing is to learn to rule over oneself."   Goethe (1749-1832)

"It is at the great and solemn crisis, decisive of our reputation with others, and yet more with ourselves, that we choose in defiance of what is conventionally called a motive, and the absence of any tangible reason is the more striking the deeper our freedom goes."   Henri   Bergson (1859-1941): "Time and Free Will"

"Be not the slave of your own past. Plunge into the sublime seas, dive deep and swim far, so you shall come back with self-respect, with new power, with an advanced experience that shall explain and overlook the old." Ralph Waldo Emerson (1803-1882)

"A foolish consistency is the hobgoblin of little minds, adored by little statesmen and philosophers and divines. With consistency a great soul has simply nothing to do. He may as well concern himself with his shadow on the wall. Speak what you think now in hard words and tomorrow speak what tomorrow thinks in hard words again, though it contradict every thing you said today.   Ralph Waldo Emerson (1803-1882): "Self Reliance"

"It is easy in the world to live after the world's opinion; it is easy in solitude to live after our own; but the great man is he who in the midst of the crowd keeps with perfect sweetness the independence of solitude." Ralph Waldo Emerson (1803-1882): "Self Reliance"

"The spirit of Man is nomad, his blood Bedouin, and love is the aboriginal tracker on the faded desert spoor of his lost self; and so I came to live my life not by conscious plan or prearranged design but as someone following the flight of a bird."   Laurens van der Post (1906-1996

"It matters not how strait the gate, How charged with punishment the scroll, I am the master of my fate: I am the captain of my soul.   W . E . Henley (1849-1903): from "Invictus"

"Lord, when I am wrong make me willing to change. When I am right, make me easier to live with."   Desmond Tutu (Contemporary)

"The great enemy of clear language is insincerity. If thought corrupts language, language can also corrupt thought."   George Orwell (1903-1950): "Politics and the English Language"

"Good writers are those who keep the language efficient. That is to say, keep it accurate, keep it clear."   Ezra Pound (1884-1972)

"Free yourself from whatever is superfluous to yourself." Goethe   (1742-1832)

"The great thing in this world is not so much where we stand, as in what direction we are moving."   Oliver Wendell Holmes (1841-1935)

"The despotism of custom is everywhere the standing hindrance to human achievement."   John Stuart Mill (1800-1873)

"Our main business is not to see what lies dimly at a distance but to do what lies clearly at hand."   Thomas Carlyle (1795-1881)

Of Work

"Everything in which man seriously interests himself stretches out to infinity; against this his only weapon is unremitting industry."   Goethe (1749-1832)

"The big differences between individuals are not in their abilities, but in their willingness to work."   Charles Darwin (1809-1882)

"The three great essentials to achieve anything worthwhile are first, hard work; second sticking to it; third commonsense."   Thomas Eddison (1847-1931)

"Singleness of purpose is one of the chief essentials for success in life."
John D. Rockefeller (1839-1937)

"True wisdom, in general, lies in energetic determination."
Napoleon (1769-1821)

"The secret of success in life is for a man to be ready for his opportunity when it comes."   Benjamin Disraeli (1804-1881)

And John Paul Getty (1892-1975), when asked what the secret of his success was, replied: "Get up early, work hard, and then strike oil."

"The boldest measures are the safest."   William Pitt (1759-1806)

"What you can do, or dream you can, begin it. Boldness has genius, power and magic in it."   Goethe (1749-1832)

"Knowledge we ask not; Knowledge thou hast lent, But Lord, the Will there lies our bitter need, Help us to build above the deep intent, the Deed, the Deed."   John Drinkwater (1749-1832)

"The men whom I have seen succeed best in life have always been cheerful and hopeful men, who went about their business with a smile on their faces, and took changes and chances of this mortal life like men facing rough and smooth alike as it came."   Charles Kingsley (1819-1915)

"Adventure, as they call it, isn't an evasion, but a quest. A break in the established order is never the work of chance; it is the outcome of a man's resolve to turn life to account." André Malraux (1901-1976): "The Royal Way"

The hero "is a man of action rather than thought and lives by a personal code of honour that admits to no qualification. His responses are usually instinctive, predictable, and inevitable. He accepts challenge and sometimes even courts disaster."   Oxford English Dictionary, 2nd Edition

Of Surgery and Education
"Men are men before they are lawyers or physicians or manufacturers; and if you make them capable and sensible men they will make themselves capable and sensible lawyers and physicians."

John Stuart Mill (1806-1873): Inaugural Address to St. Andrew's University 1867

"Only those who have the patience to do simple things perfectly will acquire the skill to do difficult things easily."   Johan Schiller (1759-1805)

However, the former quote from Schiller should be balanced against that ancient German proverb: "All skill and daring may come to naught if an angel pisses in the flintlock of your musket!"

"Be even tempered in success and failure, for it is this evenness of temper which is meant by yoga."   The Bhagavad Gita

"It is the surgeon's duty to tranquillise the temper, to beget cheerfulness and to impart confidence of recovery. Some medical practitioners are so cold and cheerless as to damp every hope; whilst others inspire confidence of recovery. It is your duty therefore to support hope, to preserve tranquillity and to inspire cheerfulness, even when you are doubtful of the issue." Sir Astley Cooper (1768-1841), Surgeon to Guy's Hospital

"Poor is the pupil who does not outshine his master." And "Education is the best provision for the journey to old age."   Aristotle (384-322 BC)

"The great secret of success is to go through life as a man who never gets used up. That is possible for him who never argues and strives too much with men and facts, but in all experiences retires upon himself, and looks for the ultimate source of things in himself."   Albert Schweitzer (1875-1965)

"Knowledge and wisdom, far from being one, have oft-times no connection. Knowledge dwells in heads replete with thoughts of other men; Wisdom in minds attentive of their own. Knowledge is proud that he has learned so much. Wisdom is humble that he knows not more."   William Cowper (1731-1800)

"We must always remember it is the balance of evidence that determines diagnosis. Remember that also in practical life in dealing with patients, the habit of discerning the probability and acting decisively is all important. Nothing is so necessary to every practitioner as the confidence of his patients. To gain that he must manifest some measure of confidence in himself. If you must wait before forming even a probable opinion at any rate be decided in delay. Remember decisive hesitation is far wiser than hesitating decision."   Sir William Gower (1845-1915)

Denton Cooley (b. 1920), the great Texan surgeon, on retirement: "It is better to retire one year too soon than one minute too late."

Of Happiness and Friendship

"Of all the things that wisdom provides to help one live one's life in happiness, the greatest by far is the possession of friendship."   Epicurus (341-270 BC)

"Think where Man's Glory most begins and ends
And say my Glory was I had such friends".   WB Yeats (1865 – 1939)

"If a man does not make new acquaintances as he advances through life, he will soon find himself left alone. A man, Sir, should keep his friendships in constant repair".   Samuel Johnson (1709 – 1784)

"The happy life is a life that is in harmony with its own nature." And "To be courageous, energetic, and attentive to good things of the world without being their slave is the recipe for happiness."   Seneca (4BC-65AD)

"Happiness consists in congenial occupation with a sense of progress." Goethe (1749-1832)

"If there is a sin against life, it consists not so much of despairing of life as in hoping for another life and in eluding the implacable grandeur of this one.   Albert Camus (1913-1960)

"For there's nothing fairer than when a man and a woman share their hearth together with minds that think alike.   Homer (circa 8th Century BC): "The Odyssey"

"The ideal of human relationships is a setting in which each partner, while acknowledging the need of the other, feels free to be what he or she by nature is: a relationship in which instinct as well as intellect can find expression; in which giving and taking are equal; in which each accepts the other, and I confronts Thou."   Anthony Storr (1920-2001)

"…while the wind in the chimney is calling to her, and the rain on the window is calling to him, in wild, intermittent desperate reminders that the cosmic mystery which men call happiness is not to be gained by a conspiracy of clinging bodies, but by the fraternisation of proud and lonely intelligences." John Cowper Powys (1872-1963)

INDEX

A

Abrahams, Harold 145
abu Shabaan, Dr Nasser 218
Academy of Medicine of Malaysia 154
Acheson, Roy 106
Acheson, Sir Donald 151
Adams, Aileen 152, 171
Adams, Chris 79
Addenbrooke, John 180
Addenbrooke's Hospital 89, 150, 180
Addington Palace 9, 40, 45
Alabaster, Margaret 87
Ann 72, 74, 77, 80, 84, 85, 116, 118,
        140, 142, 150, 153, 155, 157,
        168, 170, 172, 175, 176, 181,
        197, 198, 208, 209, 210, 228
Arthur 43, 84, 85, 202, 206, 208, 209,
        229, 230
Association of Surgeons of India 156
Atkins, Sir Hedley 68, 167
Audit Commission v, 195, 201, 202
Auger, Dave 52
Aunt Doreen (Doreen) 17, 41, 67, 71

B

Bahnson, Hank 172
Bailey, Alan 119
Baker, Charles (Dr Baker) 67, 69
Baltistan 171
Bannister, Roger 227
Barlow, Andrew 101, 102
Barnard, Christiaan (Chris Barnard)
        73, 90, 113, 193
Barnato, Barney 40
Barnes, Nick and Jo 211

Bate, Jonathan 188
Battle of Delville Wood 43
Beavis, John 215, 217, 223, 224, 225
Belcher, Jack 120
Belgian Congo 35, 36
Bell, Mary 74
Belsey, Ronald 117
Bethune, Don 97, 117, 122
Betjeman, John 174
Bewick, Michael 96
Blackwell, Barry 66
Blair, Tony 202
Blandy, John 157
Bolingbroke Hospital 68, 81
Bottomley, Virginia 151, 158
Bould, Pabby 20
Bovell, Bob 41
Bozzoli, Professor 42
Bridge, Stephen 143, 202
British Heart Foundation 104, 110
British Medical Association 125, 146,
        151, 195, 196
Brock, Sir Russell (Lord Brock, Brock)
        69, 75, 153, 162, 196
Brompton Hospital 82, 89, 125, 207
Brooksby, Ian 117
Brown, John 204, 206, 211, 222
Browse, Norman 169, 170
Buckston Browne, George 167
Buirski, Aubrey 52
Burnett, Pauline 95, 104
Burwash Landing 48, 50
Butterfield, Sir John (John Butterfield)
        100, 164, 175, 190
Buxton, Martin 106

C

Cabrol, Christian 97
Calne, Roy 91, 92, 95, 96, 98, 99, 100, 101
Campbell, Sam 32
Camus, Albert 54,231,232,236
Carmichael, James 63
Carpentier, Alain 135
Carroll, Des and Judy 85
Carter, Gwendoline 51
Castle, Keith 100, 101, 102
Caves, Philip 90, 91, 96, 105
Cementation Company 24
Chalmers, Sir Ian 218
Chapman, Roy 192
Chief Medical Officer 90, 93, 94, 98, 99, 102, 106, 151, 160
Churchill, Winston 15, 213
Clare 228
Clark, Barney 130
Clarke, Kenneth 151, 159, 161, 166
Cleland, Bill 86
Clifford Harris (Rhodesia) Ltd 25
Cockburn, Helen 78
College of Physicians and Surgeons of Pakistan 155
Concordia 172
Cooke, Stan 52, 66
Cooksey, David 201
Cooper, David 97
Copeland, Jack 127
Cordwallis School 18
Cory-Pearce, Richard 104, 108, 110
Coutielle, Jean-Paul 112
Crawhall, Mr 26, 29
Crowther, Jeremy 202,210,230
Curry, Paul 138

D

Dark, John 118, 119
Darwin, Charles 167, 231
Davies, Hywel 69
De Beers Consolidated Mines Ltd 40
de Courcy, James 218

de Hullu, Antoine and Maria 225
de Leval, Marc 140
Deputy Lieutenant of Cambridgeshire 201
Despins, Phillipe 112
Devenish, Kitty 9, 40
Dicey, Annetjie 206
Dicey, Billy 225
Dicey, David 225
Dicey, Gwen 73
Dicey, Mordaunt 72
Dicey Tom 72, 191, 204, 222
Digerness, Stan 85
Dodge, Anne 220
Doreen, Aunt 17, 41, 67, 71
Duncan, George 174
Dunn, David 195
Durham, Elaine 209

E

Eiseman, Ben 172
Elizabeth 3, 20, 24, 38, 45, 57, 144
Elliott, Alison 150
Elton, Sir Arnold 158, 159
Emerson, Ralph Waldo 56, 232
English, Alexander 3, 4, 15
English, Arthur Alexander (father) 3, 9, 15, 16, 72
English, Fred 43,46
English, Fred (Great Uncle Fred) 8, 33, 39, 40, 43, 46, 228
English, Henry 9, 43
English, William Henry 4, 5, 6
Ennals, Lord 159
Esmore, Don 112, 131, 132
Evans, David 91, 95, 105, 106, 117

F

Falcon, William 12
Fellowes, Sir Robert 157, 158
Fischer, Rheinhart 138
Fleming, Hugh 91, 92, 117
Foster, Andrew 201
Frater, Robert 73
Frossard, Jeanne 218

G

Gaddian, David 162, 163
Gairdner, Douglas 116, 117
Gaza 217, 218
Geldenhuys, Johnny 25, 26, 29
General Medical Council v, 116, 123, 140, 148, 201
Getty, Paul 169, 232
Gibbon, John 75
Gill, Roy 133
Godber, Sir George 90, 160
Goodwin, Professor John 99, 105
Gordon, Jean 4
Grabham, Tony 160
Green, Professor Colin 213
Greig, David 74
Groom, Graeme 218
Groote Schuur hospital 72
Gurdon, Jean 190
Guy's Hospital Medical School (Guy's Hospital) 41 ,45, 56, 64
Guy's Thoracic Unit 74

H

Hall, Sir Peter 188
Hanson, Lord 157
Harker, John 23
Harling, Rachel 202,230
Haslett, Michael 190
Hastillo, Andrea 126, 127
Hawthorne, Anne 3, 4
Hawthorne, Jane 4
Heart Transplantation v, 89, 125, 127
Henagan, Ann 84
Henderson, Mr 26, 29
Hepple, Bob 212
Her Majesty the Queen 135, 156
Hess, Michael 126, 127
Hill, Caroline vi
Hilton College 11, 12, 13, 14, 19, 22
Hirshorn, Joseph 47
Holdsworth, Victoria 169
Holmes-Sellors, Sir Thomas 80, 196
Hood, John 227

Hopkins, Anthony 69
Horbury, Reverend William 209
Houston, Dr George 58
Hudson, John William 22
Humana Corporation 130
Human, Jurie Johannes 8
Human, Katherine Elizabeth (Katherine) 5
Human, Matthys Gerhardus 8
Hunterian Museum 157, 169, 212
Hunterian Trustees 147
Hunter, John 142, 147, 195, 212
Huntingdon Research Centre 94, 97, 111
Hunyani Poort 26, 29

I

Ibiza 53, 54, 55
IDEALS 149, 215, 216
Irvine, Donald 201

J

James, Don 47
Jamieson, Stuart 125, 128, 211
Jaquot, Joe 49
Jarvik, Robert 130, 131
Jenkin, Patrick 103
Jenkins, Arthur 220
Jerusalem 217
Johnson-Gilbert, Ronald 120, 123, 146
Johnstone, Brian 164
Johnstone, Charles 74
Johnstone, Mary 77
Joiner, Charles 69, 70
Joklik, Frank 55, 57, 62, 133
Jones, David 131
Joubin, Franc 47
Juliet 230

K

Kabir, Mohammed 155, 215
Karp, Bob 85
Katharine 85, 182, 206, 208, 209, 210, 221, 229, 230
Kaye, Michael 128

Kennedy, Ludovic 164
Kennedy, President 77
Kerr, Findlay 117
Khyber Pass 155
Kimberley 9, 39, 40
King, Dave 212
King, Martin Luther 84
King of Malaysia 154
Kirklin, John (Dr Kirklin) 75, 84, 87, 112, 196
Kittens Club 189
Kolff, Willem 129, 131

L

Lansing, Alan 130
Lanzerac 9
Large, Steve 142, 143
Lavin, Deborah 220
Lawrie, Rex (Mr Lawrie) 67, 68, 81
le Huray, Peter 191
Lennox, Stuart 86
Leonard Cheshire Centre for Conflict Recovery 215
Leonard, Colvin 34, 36
Levin, Bernard 104
Levin, Dr Arthur (Arthur Levin) 137
Lewin, Walpole 96
Lewis, Terry 221
Leys School 202
Lillehei, Walton 75
Lincoln, Christopher 84, 89
Lister, Nancy 53
Llewellyn-Smith, Elizabeth 210
London Chest Hospital 81, 82, 84
Losman, Jacques 127, 128
Lower, Richard 90, 97
Lund, Benjamin 10, 11
Lund, Betty 146
Lund, Charles Luke 11
Lund, Mavis Eleanor (mother) 3, 12, 16, 20, 28, 53, 65, 144
Lund, Max (Uncle Max) 40
Lund, Stewart 224
Lyon, Anne 184

M

Macara, Sandy 197
Mansergh, Terence 21
Marsh, Howard 177
Marsh, Paul 204, 211, 223
Mary 86, 168, 177, 196, 199, 208, 209, 221, 224, 229
Master's Lodge 181, 191, 208
McElvey, Stuart 171, 172
McGregor, Chris 134, 211, 224
McHugh, Charles 97
McKellen, Sir Ian 188
McMaster, Paul 97, 100
Medical Aid for Palestinians (MAP) 217
Menuhin, Lord 191
Milburn, Alan 202
Mills, Frank 49, 55
Mills, Ivor 92
Milne, Judith vi, 207, 208, 209, 210, 212, 226, 228
Milne, Peter 224
Milstein, Ben 89, 91, 105, 111, 117, 118, 136, 138
Montserrat 61
Morgan, Cliff 164
Morris, Peter 106
Morse, Vice Admiral Sir Anthony 37
Mortimer, Paul 41
Mt. Kilimanjaro 219
Murley, Reginald (Reggie Murley) 146, 157, 197

N

Nashef, Sam 111
National Heart Hospital 80, 87, 94
National Heart Research Fund 101, 103
Nicholls, Professor John 213
Northwick Park Institute for Medical Research 213

O

O'Brien, Virginia 108, 109, 114
O'Donnell, Michael 164
Okavango Delta 141

Oliver, Simon 215
Ongcharit, Chawalit 112
O'Shea, Michael 159

P

Pakistan 215
Pandora 56
Paneth, Matt 82, 83, 87, 88, 89
Panorama 106
Papworth Hospital v, 89, 92, 99, 103,
        131, 174, 202, 212
Parameshwar, Jayan 174
Parish, Chris 89, 117
Parker, John 140
Parkman, Brookes 51
Parks, Sir Alan (Alan Parks) 120, 147
Parktown Preparatory School 17
Pateman, John (Mr. Pateman) 21
Pattie, Sir Geoffrey 192
Paxman, Jeremy 188
Peart, Sir Stanley (Stan Peart) 162, 213
Peckham, Sir Michael 163, 188
Petch, Michael 94, 98, 105
Phillips, Peter 81
Pinker, George 81
Plettenberg Bay 71, 72, 73, 77, 78,
        142, 191, 206, 208
Plummer, Jane 11
Popper, Karl 166
Porritt, Jonathan 164
Porritt, Lord (Arthur Porritt) 157, 164
Preliminary Proceedings Committee
        123, 124
Primary Trauma Care (PTC) 216
Prince Phillip 156
Princess Alexandra 135, 136
Princess Sirindhorn 154
Pullen, John 81

Q

Queen of Thailand 152, 153

R

Ramakrishna, Ramu 198

Rattray, David 198
Rees, Gareth 123, 147
Reitz, Bruce 111
Religa, Zbigniew 112
Rhodes, Cecil 15, 39, 74
Robb, Gale 56
Robertson, Dr 93, 100, 101
Robinson Charitable Trust 103
Robinson, David 104
Rosen, Michael 152
Ross, Barry 117
Ross, Donald 73, 76, 77, 80, 87, 90,
        98, 118, 120, 196
Ross, Keith 87, 88
Rothschild, Lord and Lady 158
Royal College of Surgeons of England
        (College of Surgeons) 59, 120,
        143, 144, 147, 150
Rubbra, Benedict 186
Rudge, Chris 96
Rudoe, Jonathan 188
Russell, Audrey 209, 224
Russell, Michael 52
Ryan, Jim 214

S

Shakeshaft, John 175, 177
Shaw, Michael 18, 19
Sheela 62, 66
Shields, Lyn 220
Shifa Hospital 218
Shumway, Norman (Dr Shumway) 90,
        96, 112, 113, 127, 196
Simpson, John 137
Simpson, Professor Keith 64
Slaney, Geoffrey 123, 147
Smartt, Sir Thomas 72
Smith, Dame Janet 124
Smith, John 163
Smith, Lord 145
Smuts, General 136
Soames, Lady 213
Soon, Professor Cham Tao 188
Spratt, Phillip 112

Spurrell, Roworth 123
Starr, Albert 83
Starzl, Tom 96
St Catharine's College v, 116, 174, 175, 186, 204
St Catherine's Monastery 204
Stewart, Evelyn 11
St Hilda's College 210
Strathern, Marilyn 210
Supple, Barry 175, 178, 179, 188
Supra-Regional Services 107
Swan, Jack 77
Swinnerton-Dyer, Sir Peter 188

T

Talbot, Ralph 207
Taylor, Martin 159
Tebbit, Norman 166
Technical Mines Consultants Ltd 46
Teck Exploration Company 46
Thatcher, Margaret 69, 111, 151, 201
The Artificial Heart v, 116
The College of Anaesthetists 152
The International Society for Heart Transplantation 125
Thesiger, Wilfred 199
Todd, Ian 145, 150
Tomkys, Sir Roger 212
Towers, Peter 158
Trafford, Tony 69, 164
Transplant Advisory Panel (TAP) 95
Transvaal Chamber of Mines 31
Tranter, Sheena 218
Treadwell, Bill 66
Trumpington, Lady 202
Tubbs, Oswald 88
Turner-Warwick, Margaret 143, 160, 170

U

UK Cardiac Surgical Register 85, 118, 119, 138
Ungava 57, 59, 60, 61, 62
University (Wits) 24, 32, 42, 169
Upjohn Lecture 141

V

Van den Berg, Van 52
Van der Merwe, Morkel 200
Varrier-Jones, Sir Pendrill 108
Venkitaroman, Professor Ashok 194
Victoria Falls 36, 205, 223
Vic Toweel 34
Vieno 50, 55
Violet (English) 7, 9, 73, 74, 77, 78
Virginia 228

W

Waldegrave, William 166, 168
Walford, Diana 161
Walker, Jim 48, 50, 51
Wallace, Governor George 84
Wallwork, John 105, 107, 108, 111, 113, 114, 133, 137, 139, 143, 174
Walton, John 125
Warner, Francis vi, 188
Warwick, Professor 78, 79
Watkins, Paul 192
Watson, Richard 79
Weissman, Freidrich 166
Wellington Hospital 123, 130, 136, 137, 145, 147
Wells, Frank 111, 131, 132, 133
Wheeldon, Dereck 132, 133
Wilkinson, Douglas 216
William 43, 86, 87, 141, 168, 203, 205, 208, 210, 229
Winston Churchill Memorial Trust 213
Wittgenstein, Ludwig 166
Wolfson Foundation 193
Woodard, Cal 51
Woodlark, Robert 180
Wright, Olive 78

Y

Yacoub, Magdi (Sir Magdi Yacoub) 103, 113, 169, 170
Yehudi Menuhin School 192
Yellowlees, Sir Henry 98, 99, 100, 106

Yukon, 48

Z

Zoellner, Frederick 194

ABOUT THE AUTHOR

Sir Terence English KBE was responsible for establishing the internationally renowned heart transplant programme at Papworth Hospital near Cambridge, where he performed Britain's first successful heart transplant in 1979.

He was born in South Africa in1932 and educated at Hilton College in Natal. He then obtained a BSc in Mining Engineering at Witwatersrand University in Johannesburg. However, shortly before completing his degree he decided he would rather be a doctor, and a small inheritance enabled him to study medicine at Guy's Hospital in London.

In 1973 Sir Terence was appointed Consultant Cardiothoracic Surgeon to Papworth and Addenbrooke's Hospitals in Cambridge. Having become aware of the good results being achieved with heart transplantation at Stanford University in California, he decided that this procedure should be made available for British patients. This led in due course to Papworth becoming a national centre for transplantation of the heart and lungs.

In 1989 he became President of The Royal College of Surgeons and was later described in the BMJ publication (1997) "With Head and Heart and Hands" as, "perhaps the best president of the medical royal colleges since the war". He was elected Master of St Catharine's College, Cambridge in 1993; Deputy Lieutenant of Cambridgeshire in 1995 and in the same year became President of the British Medical Association.

Following retirement in 2000 he has remained active and involved with a number of charities. He is currently Patron of the Primary Trauma Care Foundation and is passionate about delivering courses in trauma care to developing countries such as Pakistan and Gaza. He also enjoys participating in long 4X4 "adventure drives" to remote parts of the world.

Lightning Source UK Ltd.
Milton Keynes UK
172242UK00001B/7/P